T0358858

Neuroma, Neural Interface, and Prosthetics

Editors

PAUL S. CEDERNA
THEODORE A. KUNG

HAND CLINICS

www.hand.theclinics.com

Consulting Editor
KEVIN C. CHUNG

August 2021 • Volume 37 • Number 3

ELSEVIER

1600 John F. Kennedy Boulevard • Suite 1800 • Philadelphia, Pennsylvania, 19103-2899

http://www.theclinics.com

HAND CLINICS Volume 37, Number 3
August 2021 ISSN 0749-0712, ISBN-13: 978-0-323-79455-8

Editor: Lauren Boyle
Developmental Editor: Arlene B. Campos

Hand Clinics (ISSN 0749-0712) is published quarterly by Elsevier Inc., 360 Park Avenue South, New York, NY 10010-1710. Months of publication are February, May, August, and November. Business and Editorial Offices: 1600 John F. Kennedy Blvd., Ste. 1800, Philadelphia, PA 19103-2899. Customer Service Office: 3251 Riverport Lane, Maryland Heights, MO 63043. Periodicals postage paid at New York, NY and at additional mailing offices. Subscription price is $439.00 per year (domestic individuals), $1039.00 per year (domestic institutions), $100.00 per year (domestic students/residents), $501.00 per year (Canadian individuals), $1086.00 per year (Canadian institutions), $562.00 per year (international individuals), $1086.00 per year (international institutions), $256.00 (international students/residents), and $100.00 (Canadian students/residents). Foreign air speed delivery is included in all *Clinics* subscription prices. All prices are subject to change without notice. **POSTMASTER:** Send address changes to *Hand Clinics*, Elsevier Health Sciences Division, Subscription Customer Service, 3251 Riverport Lane, Maryland Heights, MO 63043. Customer Service (orders, claims, online, change of address): Elsevier Health Sciences Division, Subscription **Customer Service, 3251 Riverport Lane, Maryland Heights, MO 63043. Tel: 1-800-654-2452 (U.S. and Canada); 314-447-8871 (outside U.S. and Canada). Fax: 314-447-8029. E-mail: journalscustomerservice-usa@elsevier.com (for print support); journalsonlinesupport-usa@elsevier.com (for online support).**

Reprints. For copies of 100 or more of articles in this publication, please contact the Commercial Reprints Department, Elsevier Inc., 360 Park Avenue South, New York, New York 10010-1710. Tel.: 212-633-3874; Fax: 212-633-3820; E-mail: reprints@elsevier.com.

Hand Clinics is covered in *MEDLINE/PubMed (Index Medicus), Current Contents/Clinical Medicine, EMBASE/Excerpta Medica,* and *ISI/BIOMED.*

Contributors

CONSULTING EDITOR

KEVIN C. CHUNG, MD, MS
Charles B. G. de Nancrede Professor of
Surgery, Professor of Plastic Surgery and
Orthopaedic Surgery, Chief of Hand Surgery,
Michigan Medicine, The University of Michigan
Health System, University of Michigan
Comprehensive Hand Center, Assistant Dean
for Faculty Affairs, Associate Director of Global
REACH, University of Michigan Medical
School, Ann Arbor, Michigan, USA

EDITORS

PAUL S. CEDERNA, MD
Professor of Plastic Surgery and Biomedical
Engineering, Chief, Section of Plastic Surgery,
Robert Oneal Professor of Plastic Surgery,
Departments of Surgery and Biomedical
Engineering, University of Michigan, Ann Arbor,
Michigan, USA

THEODORE A. KUNG, MD
Associate Professor, Section of Plastic
Surgery, Clinical Assistant Professor,
Department of Surgery, University of Michigan,
Ann Arbor, Michigan, USA

AUTHORS

OSKAR C. ASZMANN, MD, PhD
Clinical Laboratory for Bionic Extremity
Reconstruction, Division of Plastic and
Reconstructive Surgery, Department of
Surgery, Medical University of Vienna, Vienna,
Austria

KONSTANTIN D. BERGMEISTER, MD, PhD
Clinical Laboratory for Bionic Extremity
Reconstruction, Division of Plastic and
Reconstructive Surgery, Department of
Surgery, Medical University of Vienna, Vienna,
Austria; Department of Plastic, Reconstructive
and Aesthetic Surgery, University Hospital St.
Poelten, St. Poelten, Austria

DAVID L. BROWN, MD
Section of Plastic Surgery, Department of
Surgery, University of Michigan Medical
School, Ann Arbor, Michigan, USA

MATTHEW J. CARTY, MD
Division of Plastic Surgery, Brigham and
Women's Hospital, Boston, Massachusetts,
USA

PAUL S. CEDERNA, MD
Professor of Plastic Surgery and Biomedical
Engineering, Chief, Section of Plastic Surgery,
Robert Oneal Professor of Plastic Surgery,
Departments of Surgery and Biomedical
Engineering, University of Michigan, Ann Arbor,
Michigan, USA

JONATHAN CHENG, MD, FACS
Professor and Chief of Pediatric Hand,
Peripheral Nerve, Microvascular Surgery,
Department of Plastic Surgery, The University
of Texas Southwestern Medical Center, Dallas,
Texas, USA

CYNTHIA A. CHESTEK, PhD
Associate Professor, Department of
Biomedical Engineering, Robotics Institute,
Department of Electrical Engineering and
Computer Science, Neuroscience Graduate
Program, University of Michigan, Ann Arbor,
Michigan, USA

KEVIN C. CHUNG, MD, MS
Charles B. G. de Nancrede Professor of
Surgery, Professor of Plastic Surgery and
Orthopaedic Surgery, Chief of Hand Surgery,
Michigan Medicine, The University of Michigan
Health System, University of Michigan
Comprehensive Hand Center, Assistant Dean
for Faculty Affairs, Associate Director of Global
REACH, University of Michigan Medical
School, Ann Arbor, Michigan, USA

ALICIA DAVIS, CPO
University of Michigan Orthotics and
Prosthetics Center, Ann Arbor, Michigan, USA

GREGORY A. DUMANIAN, MD
Orion H. and Lucille W. Stuteville Professor of
Plastic and Reconstructive Surgery and Chief
of Plastic Surgery, Division of Plastic and
Reconstructive Surgery, Department of
Surgery, Northwestern University Feinberg
School of Medicine, Chicago, Illinois, USA

SUSANNAH M. ENGDAHL, PhD
Department of Bioengineering, George Mason
University, Fairfax, Virginia, USA

MEGAN E. FRACOL, MD
Division of Plastic and Reconstructive Surgery,
Department of Surgery, Northwestern
University Feinberg School of Medicine,
Chicago, Illinois, USA

RAYMOND GLENN GASTON, MD
Reconstructive Center for Lost Limbs,
OrthoCarolina Hand Center, Department of
Orthopaedic Surgery, Atrium Healthcare,
Charlotte, North Carolina, USA

DEANNA H. GATES, PhD
School of Kinesiology, University of Michigan,
Ann Arbor, Michigan, USA

ANDREW JORDAN GRIER, MD
Hand Surgery Fellow, OrthoCarolina Hand
Center, Charlotte, North Carolina, USA

SARAH E. HART, MD
Section of Plastic Surgery, Department of
Surgery, University of Michigan Medical
School, Ann Arbor, Michigan, USA

HUGH M. HERR, PhD
Center for Extreme Bionics, MIT Media Lab,
Massachusetts Institute of Technology,
Cambridge, Massachusetts, USA

BENJAMIN W. HOYT, MD
Walter Reed Department of Orthopedic
Surgery, Walter Reed National Military Medical
Center, Bethesda, Maryland, USA

LINDSAY E. JANES, MD
Division of Plastic and Reconstructive Surgery,
Department of Surgery, Northwestern
University Feinberg School of Medicine,
Chicago, Illinois, USA

DENNIS S. KAO, MD
Department of Surgery, University of
Washington, Seattle, Washington, USA

EDWARD KEEFER, PhD
CEO, Nerves Incorporated, Dallas, Texas, USA

JASON H. KO, MD, MBA
Associate Professor, Division of Plastic and
Reconstructive Surgery, Departments of
Surgery and Orthopaedic Surgery,
Northwestern University Feinberg School of
Medicine, Chicago, Illinois, USA

NISHANT GANESH KUMAR, MD
Section of Plastic Surgery, Department of
Surgery, University of Michigan, Ann Arbor,
Michigan, USA

THEODORE A. KUNG, MD
Associate Professor, Section of Plastic
Surgery, Clinical Assistant Professor,
Department of Surgery, University of Michigan,
Ann Arbor, Michigan, USA

YUSHA LIU, MD, PhD
Department of Surgery, University of
Washington, Seattle, Washington, USA

BRYAN J. LOEFFLER, MD
Reconstructive Center for Lost Limbs,
OrthoCarolina Hand Center, Department of
Orthopaedic Surgery, Atrium Healthcare,
Charlotte, North Carolina, USA

CYNTHIA K. OVERSTREET, PhD
Research Engineer, Nerves Incorporated, Dallas, Texas, USA

BENJAMIN K. POTTER, MD, FACS
Department Chair, USU Department of Surgery, Director of Surgery, Walter Reed National Military Medical Center, Bethesda, Maryland, USA

STEFAN SALMINGER, MD, PhD
Clinical Laboratory for Bionic Extremity Reconstruction, Division of Plastic and Reconstructive Surgery, Department of Surgery, Medical University of Vienna, Vienna, Austria

JASON M. SOUZA, MD, FACS
Associate Professor, Department of Plastic Surgery, Director, Advanced Amputation Program, The Ohio State University, Columbus, Ohio, USA

BRIAN W. STARR, MD
Section of Plastic Surgery, University of Cincinnati Medical Center, Cincinnati, Ohio, USA

ALEX K. VASKOV, PhD
Research Fellow, Department of Biomedical Engineering, Robotics Institute, University of Michigan, Ann Arbor, Michigan, USA

ZHI YANG, PhD
Associate Professor, Department of Biomedical Engineering, University of Minnesota, Minneapolis, Minnesota, USA

Contents

Symptomatic neuromas and chronic neuropathic pain are significant problems
affecting patients' quality of life and independence that are challenging to treat.
These symptoms are due to structural and functional changes that occur peripherally within neuromas, as well as alterations that occur centrally within the brain and
spinal cord. A multimodal approach is most effective, with goals to minimize opioid
use, to capitalize on the synergistic effects of nonopioid medications and to explore
potential benefits of novel adjunctive treatments.

With the development of newer techniques for symptomatic neuroma treatment,
such as regenerative peripheral nerve interface and targeted muscle reinnervation,
transposition and coverage techniques often have been referred to as "passive techniques." In spite of its negative connotation, these passive techniques yield positive
results in a majority of patients treated. The experienced surgeon has more options
than ever before in the prevention and management of problematic neuromas. Critical appraisal of the current literature reveals no single, optimal standard of care.
Instead, surgeons have a plethora of useful techniques that can be implemented
on a case-by-case basis to optimize outcomes.

Targeted muscle reinnervation (TMR) is the surgical rerouting of severed nerve endings to nearby expendable motor nerve branches. These nerve transfers provide a
pathway for axonal growth, limiting the amputated nerve ends' disorganized attempt
at regeneration that leads to neuroma formation. In the amputee population, TMR is
successful in the treatment and prevention of chronic phantom limb pain and residual limb pain. In the nonamputee population, applications of TMR are ever expand-
ing in the treatment of chronic neuroma pain owing to trauma, compression, or
surgery. This article reviews the indications for TMR, preoperative evaluation, and
various surgical techniques.

A neuroma occurs when a regenerating transected peripheral nerve has no distal
target to reinnervate. This situation can result in a hypersensitive free nerve ending
that causes debilitating pain to affected patients. No techniques to treat symptomatic neuromas have shown consistent results. One novel physiologic solution is the

regenerative peripheral nerve interface (RPNI). RPNI consists of a transected peripheral nerve that is implanted into an autologous free skeletal muscle graft. Early clinical studies have shown promising results in the use of RPNIs to treat and prevent symptomatic neuromas. This review article describes the rationale behind the success of RPNIs and its clinical applications.

In this article, the authors propose a strategy to manage and prevent symptomatic neuromas using a combination of nerve interface approaches. By using a reconstructive paradigm, these procedures provide the components integral to organized nerve regeneration, conferring both improvements in pain and potential for myoelectric control of prostheses in the future. Given the lack of evidence at this point indicating the advantage of any single nerve interface procedure, the authors propose a management approach that maximizes physiologic restoration while limiting morbidity where possible.

Chronic pain is a significant health care problem. Many patients' pain can be linked to a neuropathic origin, diagnosed with a thorough history and physical examination, and confirmed with a diagnostic nerve block. There are new procedures designed to address neuropathic pain from symptomatic neuromas by providing physiologic targets for regenerating axons following neurectomy. Dermal wrapping of the end of a sensory nerve following transection, a technique called dermatosensory peripheral nerve interface, may provide an optimal environment to prevent neuroma pain and reduce chronic neuropathic pain.

Brain-machine interfaces (BMI) are being developed to restore upper limb function for persons with spinal cord injury or other motor degenerative conditions. BMI and implantable sensors for myoelectric prostheses directly extract information from the central or peripheral nervous system to provide users with high fidelity control of their prosthetic device. Control algorithms have been highly transferable between the 2 technologies but also face common issues. In this review of the current state of the art in each field, the authors point out similarities and differences between the 2 technologies that may guide the implementation of common solutions to these challenges.

 Video content accompanies this article at http://www.hand.theclinics.com.

Multichannel longitudinal intrafascicular electrode (LIFE) interfaces provide optimized balance of invasiveness and stability for chronic sensory stimulation and motor recording/decoding of peripheral nerve signals. Using a fascicle-specific targeting (FAST)-LIFE approach, where electrodes are individually placed within discrete sensory- and motor-related fascicular subdivisions of the residual ulnar and/or median nerves in an amputated upper limb, FAST-LIFE interfacing can provide discernment of motor intent for individual digit control of a robotic hand, and restoration of touch- and movement-related sensory feedback. The authors describe their findings from clinical studies performed with 6 human amputee trials using FAST-LIFE interfacing of the residual upper limb.

Targeted muscle reinnervation (TMR) is a surgical procedure, whereby nerves without muscle targets after extremity amputation are transferred to residual stump muscles. Thereby, the control of prosthesis is improved by increasing the number of independent muscle signals. The authors describe indications for TMR to improve prosthetic control and present standard nerve transfer matrices suitable for transhumeral and glenohumeral amputees. In addition, the perioperative procedure is described, including preoperative testing, surgical approach, and postoperative rehabilitation. Based on recent neurophysiological insights and technological advances, they present an outlook into the future of prosthetic control combining TMR and implantable electromyographic technology.

 Video content accompanies this article at http://www.hand.theclinics.com.

The quest to find the ideal prosthetic device interface that enables intuitive control has motivated several recent innovations. Although current prosthetic device control strategies have advanced the field of neuroprosthetic control, they are limited in their ability to generate reliable, stable, and specific signals to replicate the complex movements of the upper extremity. The regenerative peripheral nerve interface (RPNI) is a promising solution to enhance prosthetic device control. This article describes the development of RPNIs and summarizes its successful use in the control of advanced prosthetic devices in patients with upper extremity amputations.

The agonist-antagonist myoneural interface is a novel surgical construct and neural interfacing approach designed to augment volitional control of adapted prostheses, preserve proprioception, and prevent limb atrophy in the setting of limb amputation.

 Video content accompanies this article at http://www.hand.theclinics.com.

For those patients with partial hand level amputation who would benefit from myoelectric prosthetic digits for enhanced prehensile function, the Starfish Procedure provides muscle transfers, which allow for the generation of intuitively controlled electromyographic signals for individual digital control with minimal myoelectric cross-talk. Thoughtful preoperative planning allows for creation of multiple sources of high-quality myoelectric signal in a single operation, which does not require microsurgery, providing for wide applicability to hand surgeons of all backgrounds.

Despite the numerous prosthetic hand designs that are commercially available, people with upper limb loss still frequently report dissatisfaction and abandonment. Over the past decade there have been numerous advances in prosthetic design, control, sensation, and device attachment. Each offers the potential to enhance function and satisfaction, but most come at high costs and involve surgical risks. Here, we discuss potential barriers and solutions to promote the widespread use of novel prosthetic technology. With appropriate reimbursement, multidisciplinary care teams, device-specific rehabilitation, and patient and clinician education, such technology has the potential to revolutionize the field and improve patient outcomes.

HAND CLINICS

SERIES OF RELATED INTEREST:

Clinics in Plastic Surgery
https://www.plasticsurgery.theclinics.com/

Orthopedic Clinics of North America
https://www.orthopedic.theclinics.com/

Physical Medicine and Rehabilitation Clinics of North America
https://www.pmr.theclinics.com/

THE CLINICS ARE AVAILABLE ONLINE!
Access your subscription at:
www.theclinics.com

Preface

Neuroma, Neural Interface, and Prosthetics

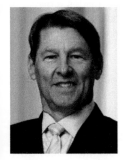 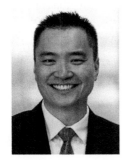

Paul S. Cederna, MD   Theodore A. Kung, MD

Editors

There are over 37 million people worldwide living with limb loss. In the United States alone, there are over 1.7 million people, with 185,000 new amputations each year. This is an incredible number of people who have sustained devastating loss of a limb, which can lead to chronic pain, inability to be gainfully employed, and even an inability to perform the simplest activities of daily living. For centuries, engineers, scientists, and physicians have attempted to improve quality of life and restore function following limb loss with a variety of static and dynamic prosthetic devices, novel interfaces, and creative surgical approaches. However, none of these interventions have come close to restoring the native functions lost following an amputation. Extending the capabilities of humans following upper and lower extremity amputations is critical to restoring form, function, and emotional well-being. We must be able to move beyond the "current state" of prosthetic rehabilitation to the point of widespread adoption of useful, scalable, and practical technology. This transition will require fundamentally new science and applications. Optimally, the human "client" should be pain free and able to connect to "host" technologies for a high-performance, multiple degree-of-freedom prosthetic device with sufficient fidelity to allow fine motor control to play the piano or to perform surgery. A closely coordinated mix of new theories and algorithms derived from our current research efforts, together with novel devices and methods from microsystems and tissue engineering, is needed to tie together the disparate threads of contemporary

peripheral nerve interface research and bring us closer to realizing the potential of tomorrow. We have made incredible progress to date but are excited about moving the technology further to make it available to the millions of people suffering from limb loss.

We are excited to provide you with this series of thoughtful and exciting articles in *Hand Clinics*: Neuroma, Neural Interface, and Prosthetics. In this issue, we have assembled the world's experts on the management of neuroma pain, residual limb pain, central and peripheral neural interface technologies, prosthetic control, and sensory feedback. We take a deep dive into better understanding the mechanisms behind residual limb pain, the traditional approaches to management, and some of the novel techniques to improve the quality of pain management. This series of outstanding articles describe all the newest and most innovative approaches to provide patients with a pain-free residual limb, which will provide them with opportunity for optimal functional restoration with prosthetic rehabilitation.

Once a patient has a pain-free residual limb following amputation, the next goal is to provide a fully integrated, bidirectional interface capable of restoring realistic and intuitive prosthetic function. For decades, we have been trying to develop interface technologies to facilitate the transmission of human motor commands to a prosthetic limb. Although robotic technology has advanced significantly in the past few decades, interface technologies have not yet kept pace. In this issue, we present recent, novel, and innovative

Hand Clin 37 (2021) xiii–xiv
https://doi.org/10.1016/j.hcl.2021.05.001
0749-0712/21/© 2021 Published by Elsevier Inc.

approaches that have demonstrated very exciting outcomes for enhanced, multifunctional prosthetic performance and bidirectional information exchange between a prosthetic device and the patient. This is not simply a discussion of a novel new engineering device but in many cases involves a paradigm shift in thinking about how to harness signals from the human body for control of the device. We discuss various brain machine interfaces to harness motor cortical signals for prosthetic control and delve into a series of diverse and creative peripheral nerve interface technologies that seek to provide a long-term, stable interface for prosthetic control. Importantly, optimal prosthetic rehabilitation not just is dependent on high-fidelity motor control, but also requires sensory feedback for intuitive motor function and prosthetic embodiment. Sensory feedback in a number of different forms is discussed as well, including a view into the potential future state.

Last, it is well known that the currently available prosthetic designs are suboptimal, with a high degree of dissatisfaction and abandonment among amputation patients. Each of the commercially available devices offers various potential benefits, but most do not accomplish the essential goal of providing naturalistic function to replace a missing limb. In this issue, we discuss the potential barriers and provide solutions to improve functional restoration with prosthetic rehabilitation through the adoption of novel prosthetic technologies. This series of articles demonstrates the dramatic advances made in recent years, illustrates how those advances have revolutionized the field of amputation rehabilitation, and provides a glimpse into the future where prosthetic devices are naturalistic in form and function and are adopted as the patient's own limb.

Paul S. Cederna, MD
Section of Plastic Surgery
University of Michigan
2130 Taubman Center
1500 East Medical Center Drive
Ann Arbor, MI 48109, USA

Theodore A. Kung, MD
Section of Plastic Surgery
University of Michigan
2130 Taubman Center
1500 East Medical Center Drive
Ann Arbor, MI 48109, USA

E-mail addresses:
cederna@umich.edu (P.S. Cederna)
thekung@umich.edu (T.A. Kung)

Nonsurgical Approaches to Neuroma Management

Yusha Liu, MD, PhD, Dennis S. Kao, MD*

KEYWORDS

- Neuropathic pain • Transcutaneous electrical nerve stimulation (TENS) • Gabapentin • Pregabalin
- Amitriptyline • Botox • Duloxetine • Magnesium

KEY POINTS

- Management of chronic neuroma/neuropathic pain requires a multimodal approach to address the complex factors that contribute to the experience of pain.
- Neuromodulators, such as gabapentin and pregabalin, are the recommended first-line medications for managing chronic neuropathic pain.
- Opioids are considered second-line medications for managing chronic neuropathic pain due to the development of tolerance, increased risk of dependence, and potential for respiratory suppression.
- Adjunctive treatments should be considered, including topical and injection medications such as lidocaine, capsaicin, and Botox, as well as nonpharmacologic methods such as mirror therapy and transcutaneous electrical nerve stimulation.

INTRODUCTION

Neuropathic pain continues to be a significant problem in the United States, with health care costs for patients afflicted with neuropathic pain being 3 times higher than a matched control group.[1] Neuropathic pain is difficult to treat effectively, with only a low percentage of patients experiencing satisfactory pain reduction from any one single intervention.[2] Therefore, a multimodal approach is recommended to maximize the synergistic effects of different combinations of medications targeting distinct pathways, while minimizing side effects.

Neuromas can form after peripheral nerve injury or transection. When the nerve is completely transected, an end neuroma forms as a result of the regenerative effort of the peripheral nerve via axonal sprouting. When a nerve is only partial transected or crushed, a neuroma-in-continuity may form. Although many neuromas are asymptomatic, it has been estimated that 13% to 32% of amputees are afflicted by symptomatic neuromas, causing pain and limiting prosthetic use.[3]

Spontaneous nerve activity in the absence of external stimuli may occur in neuromas, thus leading to generation of pain sensation in the absence of stimuli. In addition, neuromas can also have reduced excitation thresholds, making them extremely sensitive to pressure or external stimuli.[4] The reduced excitation thresholds are due to changes in the expression or function of various ion channels, resulting in hyperexcitability of nerve endings.[5] For example, changes in these ion channels are individually sufficient to cause hyperexcitability in somatosensory neurons. Therapy focused on targeting one specific ion channel tend not to be effective, as other channels can still cause hyperexcitability. These changes can also lead to hyperalgesia or allodynia. Consequently, multimodal therapeutic interventions are necessary to address the multifactorial mechanisms underlying pain.

In addition to the alterations observed in peripheral nerves, persistent afferent pain signals induce changes in the central nervous system, including changes in dorsal root ganglion and cortical reorganization. The degree of cortical reorganization

Department of Surgery, University of Washington, 325 9th Avenue, 7 CT 70, MS 359796, Seattle, WA 98104, USA
* Corresponding author.
E-mail address: dsjkao@uw.edu

Hand Clin 37 (2021) 323–333
https://doi.org/10.1016/j.hcl.2021.04.001

has been shown to be associated with increased pain intensity.[6] Therapies targeting the centralization of pain also demonstrate efficacy.

SYSTEMIC/ORAL THERAPIES

Multiple classes of oral medications have been studied in the treatment of neuroma and neuropathic pain. A summary of treatment regimens is outlined in **Table 1**.

Opioids

Opioids have been used to alleviate pain as early as 3400 BC, acting on receptors that are primarily found in the central and peripheral nervous systems, as well as the gastrointestinal tract. There are 3 major subtypes: μ-opioid receptor, δ-opioid receptor, and κ-opioid receptor. Activation of these receptors lead to a constellation of physiologic manifestations, including analgesia, respiratory depression, immunosuppression, nausea, constipation, sedation, and euphoria.[7–9]

Opioids are effective in reducing neuropathic pain for an intermediate duration of less than 12 weeks; however, despite having clinically meaningful reductions in pain levels of up to 50%, most patients do not experience improvement in many aspects of emotional or physical functioning as assessed by validated questionnaires.[10]

Chronic use of opioids may lead to opioid tolerance via receptor desensitization and downregulation such that higher doses are required over time to achieve the same level of pain relief.[11,12] However, as the dose of opioid increases, the risk of respiratory depression also increases, but without the proportional increase in pain relief. Consequently, using opioids as the sole treatment of chronic neuropathic pain is not recommended, as potential side effects outweigh therapeutic benefits. In addition, chronic exposure to opioid can paradoxically lead to hyperalgesia.[13]

With exception of cases involving cancer-related pain or palliative and end-of-life care, the current Centers for Disease Control and Prevention (CDC) guidelines for prescribing opioids for chronic pain recommend using nonpharmacological therapy and nonopioid pharmacologic therapy, establishing realistic treatment goals for pain and function, and prescribing opioids only if the benefits outweigh risks (**Box 1**).[14]

Tramadol is unique within this class of medications; in addition to its role as a μ-opioid receptor agonist, it also serves as a serotonin and noradrenaline reuptake inhibitor (SNRI). One early study showed that tramadol may reduce phantom pain intensity[15]; however, subsequent studies have failed to show efficacy in treating neuropathic pain.[16]

Gabapentin (Neurontin)

Originally developed as an antiepileptic medication, gabapentin has been used extensively in the pharmacologic treatment of neuropathic pain.[17–21] Its main target is thought to be the α_2-δ auxiliary subunit of voltage-gated calcium channels, but its mechanism of action is not well understood.[22,23] Despite some benefit in neuropathic pain secondary to traumatic or postsurgical peripheral nerve

Table 1
Summary of first-line medications

Medication	Starting Dose	Titration	Typical Target Dose	Maximum Daily Dose
Gabapentin (Neurontin)	300 mg QHS	Increase by 300 mg every 3–5 d; first increase frequency to 300 mg TID, then increase dose	1200–2400 mg/d	3600 mg
Pregabalin (Lyrica)	75 mg QHS	Increase every 3–7 d; first increase frequency to 75 mg BID, then increase dose	300–600 mg/d	600 mg
Magnesium	400 mg daily	Increase every 3–4 d, until getting 1–2 loose bowel movements per day	As tolerated with gastrointestinal side effects	1200 mg
Vitamin C	500 mg daily	Increase as tolerated	1000 mg	1500 mg
Duloxetine (Cymbalta)	30 mg daily	Increase as tolerated after 7 d, first to 60 mg/d	60–120 mg/d	120 mg
Amitriptyline (Elavil)	10 mg or 25 mg QHS	Increase as tolerated every 3–7 d	50–100 mg nightly	150 mg

injury,[24] gabapentin has demonstrated equivocal results in several clinical trials specifically examining postamputation pain. In one randomized, double-blinded, placebo-controlled, crossover trial in 19 patients with established phantom limb pain, 6 weeks of treatment with gabapentin was found to significantly decrease pain intensity compared with placebo.[25] This positive effect on pain applied also to pediatric patients who were started on gabapentin in the acute postoperative period.[26] However, a subsequent crossover study in adults failed to show benefit for phantom limb and residual limb pain, attributed to the heterogeneity of the patient population as well as overall lower initial pain ratings.[27] Another separate study of patients with lower extremity amputations due to peripheral vascular disease showed that treatment with gabapentin during the first 30 days postoperatively did not significantly decrease phantom limb or residual limb pain compared with placebo.[28] However, an extended release formulation of gabapentin was recently shown to provide significant relief of postamputation pain with excellent tolerance.[29]

The bioavailability of gabapentin is dose dependent due to a saturable transport mechanism; for a dose of 300 mg, the bioavailability is 60% but this drops to 40% when the dose is increased to 600 mg.[30] Gabapentin is not metabolized in humans and is eliminated unchanged from the body via renal excretion with good correlation to creatinine clearance.[31] It has a serum half-life between 5 and 9 hours, therefore requiring 3 times a day dosing.

The most common side effects are somnolence, dizziness, and cognitive impairment, which may be significant enough for patients to discontinue its use.[32] These adverse effects may be mitigated by slowly increasing the dose and by initiating dose increases at nighttime. A higher dose before bedtime may have the added benefit of improving sleep. In patients who show no response to gabapentin or have intolerable side effects, therapy should be slowly weaned no faster than by 300 mg every 4 days. Withdrawal symptoms, such as sweating, tachycardia, gastrointestinal symptoms, insomnia, and irritability have been reported in patients taking daily doses as low as 500 mg for 1 month and may begin 12 hours to 7 days after discontinuation.[33,34]

Pregabalin (Lyrica)

Pregabalin is a gabapentinoid medication with similar molecular mechanisms as gabapentin but has a more favorable pharmacokinetic profile, namely excellent bioavailability due to a rapid, predictable rate of absorption that, unlike gabapentin, is dose independent.[35–37] The starting dose is often clinically effective, and because a steady state concentration may be achieved within 24 to 48 hours, uptitration may be done more quickly, allowing for earlier attainment of symptom relief. In addition, pregabalin affords the convenience of twice daily dosing. Similar to gabapentin, a higher nighttime dose may facilitate sleep, and withdrawal symptoms may be observed with abrupt cessation.

The benefits of pregabalin in the treatment of neuropathic pain have primarily been studied in the context of diabetic neuropathy and postherpetic neuralgia. In addition to pain relief, treatment seems to also improve measures of anxiety and sleep interference.[38–42] Although pregabalin has not been studied specifically for postamputation or phantom limb pain, several studies have shown promising results for pain reduction in posttraumatic neuropathic pain, such as those from peripheral nerve injuries.[43–45] Most notably, in open-label trials, pregabalin has demonstrated efficacy in refractory neuropathic pain, even in patients who have failed gabapentin.[46–49] Despite the lack of evidence specific to neuroma treatment, the positive effects of pregabalin in other clinical applications have been extrapolated and, combined with its pharmacokinetic advantages, it has become the preferred first-line medication for many physicians, particularly with the introduction of a generic formulation in 2019.

Duloxetine (Cymbalta)

Duloxetine is a serotonin and SNRI with efficacy in reducing pain associated with diabetic peripheral neuropathy, fibromyalgia, and chronic musculoskeletal pain.[50–55] One case series demonstrated improvement in phantom limb pain in 4 patients after lower extremity amputation.[56] However, randomized controlled trials specifically examining postamputation and neuroma pain are otherwise lacking for both duloxetine and a closely related SNRI, venlafaxine, which is also commonly prescribed for depression and chronic pain. Nausea is common at initiation of treatment but is often transient and improves within 1 week. There is a slight risk of bleeding and hepatic dysfunction with duloxetine and an increased risk of serotonin syndrome if combined with other medications targeting serotonergic neurotransmission.

Amitriptyline (Elavil)

Amitriptyline is a tricyclic antidepressant (TCA) that inhibits neuronal reuptake of serotonin and norepinephrine and is frequently used to treat a variety of types of chronic pain, although onset of analgesia may take many weeks.[57] For pain after amputation, one double-blinded, randomized, placebo-controlled study in 39 patients did not demonstrate any benefit of amitriptyline.[58] Other medications in the TCA family include nortriptyline, imipramine, desipramine, and doxepin but none have been studied in the context of postamputation pain. Relative contraindications for TCA use include cardiovascular disorders, as amitriptyline may increase risk of sinus tachycardia, cardiac conduction time changes, arrhythmias, myocardial infarction, and stroke.

N-Methyl-D-Aspartate Receptor Antagonists

N-methyl-D-aspartate (NMDA) receptors bind to the excitatory neurotransmitter glutamate and are involved in both nociception as well as central sensitization of pain.[59] Two NMDA antagonists are frequently used in a clinical setting: ketamine is most commonly used for analgesia in acute pain, and memantine is used for treatment of neurocognitive deficits in Alzheimer disease. Both medications are generally well tolerated by patients. Given their mechanism of action and favorable side-effect profile, there was intense interest in exploring their potential in treating postamputation pain; however, although initial studies were promising, multiple clinical trials have failed to show benefits.[60–64]

Magnesium

Although not a primary analgesic, magnesium sulfate can be used as an adjunct to enhance the analgesic actions of other medications. Magnesium can prevent the induction of central sensitization from peripheral pain stimuli by blocking NMDA receptors in a voltage-dependent manner.[65] It also functions as a calcium channel blocker and inhibits catechol release from peripheral nerve endings. In animal models, it has been shown to amplify the analgesic effects of low-dose morphine and delay morphine tolerance.[66]

Oral magnesium tablets include magnesium ascorbate, magnesium citrate, or magnesium oxide. Magnesium taken orally is a laxative and can reduce constipation side effects from several routinely used analgesics, including opioids and antidepressants. Patients may experience diarrhea at the initiation of oral magnesium, but this usually improves with time. Although generally well tolerated, magnesium may cause muscle weakness and electrocardiogram changes when serum levels are elevated. Risks and benefits of treatment must be carefully considered in patients with preexisting neuromuscular diseases or cardiac arrhythmias; in addition, because magnesium is primarily renally excreted, caution should be exercised in patients with kidney disease.

Vitamin C

Originally gaining notoriety in its association with scurvy, vitamin C serves as a cofactor for a variety of functions in the body, including neurotransmitter and peptide hormone biosynthesis.[67,68] Epidemiologic studies have shown that patients suffering from postherpetic neuralgia have lower serum vitamin C levels and administration of intravenous vitamin C leads to a reduction in pain.[69,70] Moreover, vitamin C supplementation for about 6 weeks, particularly at doses greater than 500 mg, decreases the risk of developing complex regional pain syndrome after wrist and ankle surgery.[71–73] Interestingly, vitamin C has also been shown to decrease opioid analgesic requirements following surgical procedures.[74–76] With minimal side effects accompanying these potential benefits, vitamin C supplementation should be considered in the treatment of neuroma pain.

Cannabis-Based Medicines

The recent legalization of recreational cannabis in many regions of the United States has been associated with an exponential increase in the use of cannabis-based medications, including tetrahydrocannabinol, a psychoactive agent, and cannabidiol, an antiinflammatory component of cannabis.[77] Often touted as a natural, herbal alternative to conventional pharmacologic agents, cannabinoids have gained popularity particularly in patients with chronic and neuropathic pain, and health care providers are increasingly asked about their opinions regarding these products. There are few randomized controlled clinical trials examining the efficacy of cannabinoids but a recent Cochrane review does not show significant efficacy for the treatment of neuropathic pain from various causes.[78]

THERAPIES FOR TOPICAL APPLICATION OR LOCALIZED INJECTION
Lidocaine

Injection of local anesthetics such as lidocaine into the suspected site of a neuroma or proximally along the course of the affected nerve is a useful diagnostic test commonly performed in the clinical setting.[79] Therapeutic use of lidocaine may be via creams, which require multiple applications per day, or patch, which requires only once daily application. Topical administration is very safe, as there is minimal systemic absorption and toxicity or adverse interactions with other medications, and well-tolerated, with mild skin irritation being the most common complaint.[80] In a randomized, double-blinded, placebo-controlled study, use of 5% lidocaine patches was effective in reducing pain and allodynia in patients with focal peripheral neuropathic pain with the number needed to treat being 4.4.[81] Patients continued to experience the positive benefits from lidocaine patches even with long-term use over several years.[82] Although patients with suspected neuromas were included in all of these studies, other patients with focal nerve pain such as postherpetic neuropathy were also included, which may somewhat limit the generalizability for neuroma-specific pain.

Capsaicin

Capsaicin, the active ingredient found in chili peppers, is a selective TRPV1 receptor agonist that alleviates pain through the desensitization of TRPV1 channels and defunctionalization of nociceptors.[83–85] Topical formulations with 8% capsaicin have demonstrated modest analgesic benefits for postherpetic neuralgia, diabetic neuropathy, and human immunodeficiency virus–associated neuropathy; however, these effects are thought to be limited to nociceptive sensory nerve fibers within the skin rather than analgesia through transdermal delivery to nerve fibers in deeper tissues.[86] Interestingly, in a study looking specifically at limb amputations, a single 60-minute application of an 8% capsaicin patch led to decreased stump pain and hypersensitivity with evidence of acute cortical changes in limb representation demonstrated on functional MRI.[87] A double-blinded, randomized controlled trial examining pain associated with Morton's neuroma showed that a single injection of capsaicin into the region of the neuroma reduced pain scores, improved mood, and decreased walking interference for at least 4 weeks compared with a placebo injection.[88] Despite these intriguing findings and a wealth of basic science knowledge about the TRPV1 receptor, capsaicin is not widely used in the treatment of painful neuromas.

Botulinum Toxin (Botox)

Botulinum toxin is a protein produced by anaerobic bacteria Clostridium botulinum, and of multiple subtypes, types A and B are the most common for clinical use. Botulinum toxin inhibits presynaptic release of acetylcholine at the neuromuscular junction, causing flaccid muscle paralysis. Previously, the analgesic effect of botulinum toxin was thought to be due to its facilitation of muscle relaxation[89]; however, more recent studies have implicated an alternative mechanism of analgesia, which is supported by a dissociation in the duration of pain relief compared with the duration of muscle relaxation, and this has been attributed to botulinum toxin's ability to also inhibit the release of pain mediators including substance P and glutamate.[90,91]

Early case series showed a potential benefit in the use of botulinum toxin for postamputation pain.[92–94] In a subsequent prospective, randomized, double-blinded pilot study with 14 patients, injection of 50 units per painful site resulted in improved residual limb pain for several months without an effect on phantom limb pain.[95] In addition, botulinum toxin may improve stump myoclonus and hyperhidrosis, which may improve patient comfort in their prosthetic socket.[96,97]

NONPHARMACOLOGIC THERAPIES
Graded Motor Imagery/Mirror Therapy

Graded motor imagery is a behavioral therapy that targets the cortical representation of the amputated limb, as maladaptive alterations in the somatosensory and motor areas of the brain following amputation are thought to contribute to phantom limb pain.[6,98–100] This form of therapy uses a sequence of strategies including left/right discrimination, explicit motor imagery, and mirror therapy. Of these components, mirror therapy has been studied most extensively. In this technique, a mirror is placed in front of the amputated limb, and the reflected image is that of the normal limb, such that the intact limb is superimposed on the position of the phantom limb; this gives the patient the illusion that movements of the intact limb that are observed in the mirror originate from the phantom limb and promotes favorable cortical reorganization after limb loss. After limb amputation, the brain continues to send motor commands to the missing limb but lacks the sensory feedback of limb movement, and this phenomenon of learned paralysis is theorized to contribute to phantom limb pain.[101] Several small randomized controlled trials using mirror therapy have demonstrated positive effects for patients with both upper and lower extremity amputations.[102–106] Recent developments in technology have adapted this principle into virtual reality and augmented reality platforms with similar success in pilot studies.[107–109]

Transcutaneous Electrical Nerve Stimulation

Although the main nonsurgical approach to the treatment of neuropathic pain remains pharmacologic, it is also common for patients to pursue adjunct nonpharmacological interventions (psychological or physical), such as transcutaneous electrical nerve stimulation (TENS). TENS units typically use adhesive surface electrodes applied to the skin to deliver pulsed electrical stimulation that can be modified by frequency, intensity, and duration.[110] Intensity is a critical factor in optimizing TENS efficacy; it is necessary to deliver a strong, nonpainful sensation that is titrated during treatment to maintain the intensity level.[111,112] The analgesic effect of TENS may be partially mediated by peripheral mechanisms, as pretreatment administration of a peripheral opioid receptor blocker decreased the analgesic effect of TENS.[113] TENS may also reduce pain perception through the spinal pathway via the "pain-gate" mechanism, which postulates that large diameter Aβ afferent fibers involved in touch and vibration sensation inhibit nociceptive activity in the dorsal horn of the spinal cord, leading to decreased pain perception.[114] In 1967, electrical stimulation was first demonstrated to provide pain relief in patients even half an hour after the cessation of treatment.[115] Despite several studies showing encouraging results,[104] the most recent Cochrane review did not demonstrate strong evidence for efficacy of TENS in the treatment of neuropathic pain.[116] Side effects of use are rare and include skin irritation under the electrode pads.

Transcranial Magnetic Stimulation

Transcranial magnetic stimulation (TMS) is a noninvasive technique for neuromodulation in which magnetic pulses are used to stimulate specific regions of the brain. Clinically, TMS has been most frequently used in the treatment of refractory depression. Several small studies, including one randomized controlled trial, have explored its application in phantom limb pain, with promising results showing that pain relief may last for weeks after treatment.[117–123] However, the stimulation parameters, including brain region, intensity, rate, duration, and number of sessions, varied greatly between studies; further studies are required to determine the optimal parameters and establish efficacy.

SUMMARY

The multifactorial causes of neuropathic pain pose a significant challenge to the development of effective treatments. Although different medications may alleviate certain subtypes of neuropathic pain, no one single medication or modality has demonstrated consistent efficacy in treating neuroma pain. Many of the recommendations are extrapolated from data in the treatment of other types of neuropathic pain such as diabetic neuropathy or postherpetic neuralgia. Further investigation of the use of these treatments for neuroma pain, particularly in conjunction with emerging surgical strategies, is warranted to develop a comprehensive approach to addressing neuropathic pain.

CLINICS CARE POINTS

- Structural and functional changes occur within neuromas, and these influence central alterations within the brain and spinal cord.
- Effective neuroma pain management requires a multimodal approach, potentially including various oral and topical medications, as well as nonpharmacologic therapies.

- Gabapentin or pregabalin, combined with magnesium and vitamin C, should be considered first-line medications. Opioids should be used as needed and reserved as a second-line option.
- Botox injections, topical lidocaine, topical capsaicin, graded motor imagery, and TENS may all be considered as adjunct treatments for neuropathic pain.

DISCLOSURE

The authors have nothing to disclose.

REFERENCES

1. Berger A, Dukes EM, Oster G. Clinical characteristics and economic costs of patients with painful neuropathic disorders. J Pain 2004;5(3):143–9.
2. Kalso E, Aldington DJ, Moore RA. Drugs for neuropathic pain. BMJ 2013;347:f7339.
3. Pet MA, Ko JH, Friedly JL, et al. Does targeted nerve implantation reduce neuroma pain in amputees? Clin Orthop Relat Res 2014;472(10):2991–3001.
4. Wall PD, Gutnick M. Properties of afferent nerve impulses originating from a neuroma. Nature 1974; 248(5451):740–3.
5. Ratte S, Prescott SA. Afferent hyperexcitability in neuropathic pain and the inconvenient truth about its degeneracy. Curr Opin Neurobiol 2016;36:31–7.
6. Flor H, Elbert T, Knecht S, et al. Phantom-limb pain as a perceptual correlate of cortical reorganization following arm amputation. Nature 1995;375(6531): 482–4.
7. Pattinson KT. Opioids and the control of respiration. Br J Anaesth 2008;100(6):747–58.
8. Ordaz-Sanchez I, Weber RJ, Rice KC, et al. Chemotaxis of human and rat leukocytes by the delta-selective non-peptidic opioid SNC 80. Rev Latinoam Microbiol 2003;45(1–2):16–23.
9. Feng Y, He X, Yang Y, et al. Current research on opioid receptor function. Curr Drug Targets 2012; 13(2):230–46.
10. McNicol ED, Midbari A, Eisenberg E. Opioids for neuropathic pain. Cochrane Database Syst Rev 2013;(8):CD006146.
11. Koch T, Hollt V. Role of receptor internalization in opioid tolerance and dependence. Pharmacol Ther 2008;117(2):199–206.
12. Mayer P, Hollt V. Pharmacogenetics of opioid receptors and addiction. Pharmacogenet Genomics 2006;16(1):1–7.
13. Higgins C, Smith BH, Matthews K. Evidence of opioid-induced hyperalgesia in clinical populations after chronic opioid exposure: a systematic review

and meta-analysis. Br J Anaesth 2019;122(6): e114–26.
14. Dowell D, Haegerich TM, Chou R. CDC guideline for prescribing opioids for chronic pain–United States, 2016. JAMA 2016;315(15):1624–45.
15. Wilder-Smith CH, Hill LT, Laurent S. Postamputation pain and sensory changes in treatment-naive patients: characteristics and responses to treatment with tramadol, amitriptyline, and placebo. Anesthesiology 2005;103(3):619–28.
16. Duehmke RM, Derry S, Wiffen PJ, et al. Tramadol for neuropathic pain in adults. Cochrane Database Syst Rev 2017;6:CD003726.
17. Wiffen PJ, Derry S, Bell RF, et al. Gabapentin for chronic neuropathic pain in adults. Cochrane Database Syst Rev 2017;6:CD007938.
18. Backonja M, Beydoun A, Edwards KR, et al. Gabapentin for the symptomatic treatment of painful neuropathy in patients with diabetes mellitus: a randomized controlled trial. JAMA 1998;280(21): 1831–6.
19. Rowbotham M, Harden N, Stacey B, et al. Gabapentin for the treatment of postherpetic neuralgia: a randomized controlled trial. JAMA 1998; 280(21):1837–42.
20. Rice AS, Maton S, Postherpetic Neuralgia Study G. Gabapentin in postherpetic neuralgia: a randomised, double blind, placebo controlled study. Pain 2001;94(2):215–24.
21. Serpell MG, Neuropathic pain study g. Gabapentin in neuropathic pain syndromes: a randomised, double-blind, placebo-controlled trial. Pain 2002; 99(3):557–66.
22. Kukkar A, Bali A, Singh N, et al. Implications and mechanism of action of gabapentin in neuropathic pain. Arch Pharm Res 2013;36(3):237–51.
23. Taylor CP, Gee NS, Su TZ, et al. A summary of mechanistic hypotheses of gabapentin pharmacology. Epilepsy Res 1998;29(3):233–49.
24. Gordh TE, Stubhaug A, Jensen TS, et al. Gabapentin in traumatic nerve injury pain: a randomized, double-blind, placebo-controlled, cross-over, multi-center study. Pain 2008;138(2):255–66.
25. Bone M, Critchley P, Buggy DJ. Gabapentin in postamputation phantom limb pain: a randomized, double-blind, placebo-controlled, cross-over study. Reg Anesth Pain Med 2002;27(5):481–6.
26. Wang X, Yi Y, Tang D, et al. Gabapentin as an adjuvant therapy for prevention of acute phantom-limb pain in pediatric patients undergoing amputation for malignant bone tumors: a prospective double-blind randomized controlled trial. J Pain Symptom Manage 2018;55(3):721–7.
27. Smith DG, Ehde DM, Hanley MA, et al. Efficacy of gabapentin in treating chronic phantom limb and residual limb pain. J Rehabil Res Dev 2005;42(5): 645–54.

28. Nikolajsen L, Finnerup NB, Kramp S, et al. A randomized study of the effects of gabapentin on postamputation pain. Anesthesiology 2006; 105(5):1008–15.

29. Knezevic NN, Aijaz T, Candido KD, et al. The effect of once-daily gabapentin extended release formulation in patients with postamputation pain. Front Pharmacol 2019;10:504.

30. Rose MA, Kam PC. Gabapentin: pharmacology and its use in pain management. Anaesthesia 2002;57(5):451–62.

31. Blum RA, Comstock TJ, Sica DA, et al. Pharmacokinetics of gabapentin in subjects with various degrees of renal function. Clin Pharmacol Ther 1994; 56(2):154–9.

32. Parsons B, Tive L, Huang S. Gabapentin: a pooled analysis of adverse events from three clinical trials in patients with postherpetic neuralgia. Am J Geriatr Pharmacother 2004;2(3):157–62.

33. Rosebush PI, MacQueen GM, Mazurek MF. Catatonia following gabapentin withdrawal. J Clin Psychopharmacol 1999;19(2):188–9.

34. Mersfelder TL, Nichols WH. Gabapentin: abuse, dependence, and withdrawal. Ann Pharmacother 2016;50(3):229–33.

35. Ben-Menachem E. Pregabalin pharmacology and its relevance to clinical practice. Epilepsia 2004; 45(Suppl 6):13–8.

36. Gore M, Sadosky A, Tai KS, et al. A retrospective evaluation of the use of gabapentin and pregabalin in patients with postherpetic neuralgia in usual-care settings. Clin Ther 2007;29(8): 1655–70.

37. Bockbrader HN, Wesche D, Miller R, et al. A comparison of the pharmacokinetics and pharmacodynamics of pregabalin and gabapentin. Clin Pharmacokinet 2010;49(10):661–9.

38. Dworkin RH, Corbin AE, Young JP Jr, et al. Pregabalin for the treatment of postherpetic neuralgia: a randomized, placebo-controlled trial. Neurology 2003;60(8):1274–83.

39. Lesser H, Sharma U, LaMoreaux L, et al. Pregabalin relieves symptoms of painful diabetic neuropathy: a randomized controlled trial. Neurology 2004;63(11):2104–10.

40. Freynhagen R, Strojek K, Griesing T, et al. Efficacy of pregabalin in neuropathic pain evaluated in a 12-week, randomised, double-blind, multicentre, placebo-controlled trial of flexible- and fixed-dose regimens. Pain 2005;115(3):254–63.

41. Sabatowski R, Galvez R, Cherry DA, et al. Pregabalin reduces pain and improves sleep and mood disturbances in patients with post-herpetic neuralgia: results of a randomised, placebo-controlled clinical trial. Pain 2004;109(1–2):26–35.

42. Rosenstock J, Tuchman M, LaMoreaux L, et al. Pregabalin for the treatment of painful diabetic peripheral neuropathy: a double-blind, placebo-controlled trial. Pain 2004;110(3):628–38.

43. van Seventer R, Bach FW, Toth CC, et al. Pregabalin in the treatment of post-traumatic peripheral neuropathic pain: a randomized double-blind trial. Eur J Neurol 2010;17(8):1082–9.

44. Markman J, Resnick M, Greenberg S, et al. Efficacy of pregabalin in post-traumatic peripheral neuropathic pain: a randomized, double-blind, placebo-controlled phase 3 trial. J Neurol 2018; 265(12):2815–24.

45. Jenkins TM, Smart TS, Hackman F, et al. Efficient assessment of efficacy in post-traumatic peripheral neuropathic pain patients: pregabalin in a randomized, placebo-controlled, crossover study. J Pain Res 2012;5:243–50.

46. Stacey BR, Dworkin RH, Murphy K, et al. Pregabalin in the treatment of refractory neuropathic pain: results of a 15-month open-label trial. Pain Med 2008;9(8):1202–8.

47. Navarro A, Saldana MT, Perez C, et al. Patient-reported outcomes in subjects with neuropathic pain receiving pregabalin: evidence from medical practice in primary care settings. Pain Med 2010; 11(5):719–31.

48. Freynhagen R, Grond S, Schupfer G, et al. Efficacy and safety of pregabalin in treatment refractory patients with various neuropathic pain entities in clinical routine. Int J Clin Pract 2007;61(12):1989–96.

49. Blanco Tarrio E, Galvez Mateos R, Zamorano Bayarri E, et al. Effectiveness of pregabalin as monotherapy or combination therapy for neuropathic pain in patients unresponsive to previous treatments in a Spanish primary care setting. Clin Drug Investig 2013;33(9):633–45.

50. Lunn MP, Hughes RA, Wiffen PJ. Duloxetine for treating painful neuropathy, chronic pain or fibromyalgia. Cochrane Database Syst Rev 2014;(1): CD007115.

51. Chappell AS, Desaiah D, Liu-Seifert H, et al. A double-blind, randomized, placebo-controlled study of the efficacy and safety of duloxetine for the treatment of chronic pain due to osteoarthritis of the knee. Pain Pract 2011;11(1):33–41.

52. Skljarevski V, Zhang S, Desaiah D, et al. Duloxetine versus placebo in patients with chronic low back pain: a 12-week, fixed-dose, randomized, double-blind trial. J Pain 2010;11(12): 1282–90.

53. Goldstein DJ, Lu Y, Detke MJ, et al. Duloxetine vs. placebo in patients with painful diabetic neuropathy. Pain 2005;116(1–2):109–18.

54. Raskin J, Pritchett YL, Wang F, et al. A double-blind, randomized multicenter trial comparing duloxetine with placebo in the management of diabetic peripheral neuropathic pain. Pain Med 2005;6(5): 346–56.

55. Russell IJ, Mease PJ, Smith TR, et al. Efficacy and safety of duloxetine for treatment of fibromyalgia in patients with or without major depressive disorder: Results from a 6-month, randomized, double-blind, placebo-controlled, fixed-dose trial. Pain 2008; 136(3):432–44.

56. Dalkiran M, Genc A, Dikmen B, et al. Phantom limb pain treated with Duloxetine: a case series. Klinik Psikofarmakol Bülteni 2017;26(4):409–12.

57. Moore RA, Derry S, Aldington D, et al. Amitriptyline for neuropathic pain in adults. Cochrane Database Syst Rev 2015;(7):CD008242.

58. Robinson LR, Czerniecki JM, Ehde DM, et al. Trial of amitriptyline for relief of pain in amputees: results of a randomized controlled study. Arch Phys Med Rehabil 2004;85(1):1–6.

59. Petrenko AB, Yamakura T, Baba H, et al. The role of N-methyl-D-aspartate (NMDA) receptors in pain: a review. Anesth Analg 2003;97(4):1108–16.

60. Nikolajsen L, Hansen CL, Nielsen J, et al. The effect of ketamine on phantom pain: a central neuropathic disorder maintained by peripheral input. Pain 1996;67(1):69–77.

61. Schwenkreis P, Maier C, Pleger B, et al. NMDA-mediated mechanisms in cortical excitability changes after limb amputation. Acta Neurol Scand 2003;108(3):179–84.

62. Maier C, Dertwinkel R, Mansourian N, et al. Efficacy of the NMDA-receptor antagonist memantine in patients with chronic phantom limb pain–results of a randomized double-blinded, placebo-controlled trial. Pain 2003;103(3):277–83.

63. Wiech K, Kiefer RT, Topfner S, et al. A placebo-controlled randomized crossover trial of the N-methyl-D-aspartic acid receptor antagonist, memantine, in patients with chronic phantom limb pain. Anesth Analg 2004;98(2):408–13. table of contents.

64. Nikolajsen L, Gottrup H, Kristensen AG, et al. Memantine (a N-methyl-D-aspartate receptor antagonist) in the treatment of neuropathic pain after amputation or surgery: a randomized, double-blinded, cross-over study. Anesth Analg 2000; 91(4):960–6.

65. Woolf CJ, Thompson SW. The induction and maintenance of central sensitization is dependent on N-methyl-D-aspartic acid receptor activation; implications for the treatment of post-injury pain hypersensitivity states. Pain 1991;44(3):293–9.

66. McCarthy RJ, Kroin JS, Tuman KJ, et al. Antinociceptive potentiation and attenuation of tolerance by intrathecal co-infusion of magnesium sulfate and morphine in rats. Anesth Analg 1998;86(4):830–6.

67. Carr AC, McCall C. The role of vitamin C in the treatment of pain: new insights. J Transl Med 2017;15(1):77.

68. Merkler DJ. C-terminal amidated peptides: production by the in vitro enzymatic amidation of glycine-extended peptides and the importance of the amide to bioactivity. Enzyme Microb Technol 1994;16(6):450–6.

69. Chen JY, Chang CY, Feng PH, et al. Plasma vitamin C is lower in postherpetic neuralgia patients and administration of vitamin C reduces spontaneous pain but not brush-evoked pain. Clin J Pain 2009; 25(7):562–9.

70. Schencking M, Vollbracht C, Weiss G, et al. Intravenous vitamin C in the treatment of shingles: results of a multicenter prospective cohort study. Med Sci Monit 2012;18(4):CR215–24.

71. Zollinger PE, Tuinebreijer WE, Kreis RW, et al. Effect of vitamin C on frequency of reflex sympathetic dystrophy in wrist fractures: a randomised trial. Lancet 1999;354(9195):2025–8.

72. Zollinger PE, Tuinebreijer WE, Breederveld RS, et al. Can vitamin C prevent complex regional pain syndrome in patients with wrist fractures? A randomized, controlled, multicenter dose-response study. J Bone Joint Surg Am 2007; 89(7):1424–31.

73. Besse JL, Gadeyne S, Galand-Desme S, et al. Effect of vitamin C on prevention of complex regional pain syndrome type I in foot and ankle surgery. Foot Ankle Surg 2009;15(4):179–82.

74. Jeon Y, Park JS, Moon S, et al. Effect of intravenous high dose vitamin c on postoperative pain and morphine use after laparoscopic colectomy: a randomized controlled trial. Pain Res Manag 2016; 2016:9147279.

75. Ayatollahi V, Dehghanpour Farashah S, Behdad S, et al. Effect of intravenous vitamin C on postoperative pain in uvulopalatopharyngoplasty with tonsillectomy. Clin Otolaryngol 2017;42(1):139–43.

76. Kanazi GE, El-Khatib MF, Yazbeck-Karam VG, et al. Effect of vitamin C on morphine use after laparoscopic cholecystectomy: a randomized controlled trial. Can J Anaesth 2012;59(6):538–43.

77. Hill KP. Medical marijuana for treatment of chronic pain and other medical and psychiatric problems: a clinical review. JAMA 2015;313(24):2474–83.

78. Mucke M, Phillips T, Radbruch L, et al. Cannabis-based medicines for chronic neuropathic pain in adults. Cochrane Database Syst Rev 2018;3: CD012182.

79. Arnold DMJ, Wilkens SC, Coert JH, et al. Diagnostic criteria for symptomatic neuroma. Ann Plast Surg 2019;82(4):420–7.

80. Gammaitoni AR, Alvarez NA, Galer BS. Safety and tolerability of the lidocaine patch 5%, a targeted peripheral analgesic: a review of the literature. J Clin Pharmacol 2003;43(2):111–7.

81. Meier T, Wasner G, Faust M, et al. Efficacy of lidocaine patch 5% in the treatment of focal peripheral

neuropathic pain syndromes: a randomized, double-blind, placebo-controlled study. Pain 2003;106(1–2):151–8.

82. Wilhelm IR, Tzabazis A, Likar R, et al. Long-term treatment of neuropathic pain with a 5% lidocaine medicated plaster. Eur J Anaesthesiol 2010;27(2):169–73.

83. Wong GY, Gavva NR. Therapeutic potential of vanilloid receptor TRPV1 agonists and antagonists as analgesics: Recent advances and setbacks. Brain Res Rev 2009;60(1):267–77.

84. Anand P, Bley K. Topical capsaicin for pain management: therapeutic potential and mechanisms of action of the new high-concentration capsaicin 8% patch. Br J Anaesth 2011;107(4):490–502.

85. Nolano M, Simone DA, Wendelschafer-Crabb G, et al. Topical capsaicin in humans: parallel loss of epidermal nerve fibers and pain sensation. Pain 1999;81(1–2):135–45.

86. Derry S, Rice ASC, Cole P, et al. Topical capsaicin (high concentration) for chronic neuropathic pain in adults. Cochrane Database Syst Rev 2017;(1):CD007393.

87. Privitera R, Birch R, Sinisi M, et al. Capsaicin 8% patch treatment for amputation stump and phantom limb pain: a clinical and functional MRI study. J Pain Res 2017;10:1623–34.

88. Campbell CM, Diamond E, Schmidt WK, et al. A randomized, double-blind, placebo-controlled trial of injected capsaicin for pain in Morton's neuroma. Pain 2016;157(6):1297–304.

89. Foster L, Clapp L, Erickson M, et al. Botulinum toxin A and chronic low back pain: a randomized, double-blind study. Neurology 2001;56(10):1290–3.

90. Park HJ, Lee Y, Lee J, et al. The effects of botulinum toxin A on mechanical and cold allodynia in a rat model of neuropathic pain. Can J Anaesth 2006;53(5):470–7.

91. Hehr JD, Schoenbrunner AR, Janis JE. The use of botulinum toxin in pain management: basic science and clinical applications. Plast Reconstr Surg 2020;145(3):629e–36e.

92. Jin L, Kollewe K, Krampfl K, et al. Treatment of phantom limb pain with botulinum toxin type A. Pain Med 2009;10(2):300–3.

93. Kern U, Martin C, Scheicher S, et al. Effects of botulinum toxin type B on stump pain and involuntary movements of the stump. Am J Phys Med Rehabil 2004;83(5):396–9.

94. Kern U, Martin C, Scheicher S, et al. Botulinum toxin type A influences stump pain after limb amputations. J Pain Symptom Manage 2003;26(6):1069–70.

95. Wu H, Sultana R, Taylor KB, et al. A prospective randomized double-blinded pilot study to examine the effect of botulinum toxin type A injection versus

Lidocaine/Depomedrol injection on residual and phantom limb pain: initial report. Clin J Pain 2012;28(2):108–12.

96. Charrow A, DiFazio M, Foster L, et al. Intradermal botulinum toxin type A injection effectively reduces residual limb hyperhidrosis in amputees: a case series. Arch Phys Med Rehabil 2008;89(7):1407–9.

97. Briand MM, Boudier-Reveret M, Rodrigue X, et al. A moving residual limb: botulinum toxin to the rescue. Transl Neurosci 2020;11:34–7.

98. Flor H, Nikolajsen L, Staehelin Jensen T. Phantom limb pain: a case of maladaptive CNS plasticity? Nat Rev Neurosci 2006;7(11):873–81.

99. Lotze M, Flor H, Grodd W, et al. Phantom movements and pain. An fMRI study in upper limb amputees. Brain 2001;124(Pt 11):2268–77.

100. Brunelli S, Morone G, Iosa M, et al. Efficacy of progressive muscle relaxation, mental imagery, and phantom exercise training on phantom limb: a randomized controlled trial. Arch Phys Med Rehabil 2015;96(2):181–7.

101. Ramachandran VS, Rogers-Ramachandran D. Synaesthesia in phantom limbs induced with mirrors. Proc Biol Sci 1996;263(1369):377–86.

102. Finn SB, Perry BN, Clasing JE, et al. A randomized, controlled trial of mirror therapy for upper extremity phantom limb pain in male amputees. Front Neurol 2017;8:267.

103. Chan BL, Witt R, Charrow AP, et al. Mirror therapy for phantom limb pain. N Engl J Med 2007;357(21):2206–7.

104. Tilak M, Isaac SA, Fletcher J, et al. Mirror therapy and transcutaneous electrical nerve stimulation for management of phantom limb pain in amputees - a single blinded randomized controlled trial. Physiother Res Int 2016;21(2):109–15.

105. Ol HS, Van Heng Y, Danielsson L, et al. Mirror therapy for phantom limb and stump pain: a randomized controlled clinical trial in landmine amputees in Cambodia. Scand J Pain 2018;18(4):603–10.

106. Herrador Colmenero L, Perez Marmol JM, Marti-Garcia C, et al. Effectiveness of mirror therapy, motor imagery, and virtual feedback on phantom limb pain following amputation: a systematic review. Prosthet Orthot Int 2018;42(3):288–98.

107. Perry BN, Armiger RS, Wolde M, et al. Clinical trial of the virtual integration environment to treat phantom limb pain with upper extremity amputation. Front Neurol 2018;9:770.

108. Ambron E, Miller A, Kuchenbecker KJ, et al. Immersive low-cost virtual reality treatment for phantom limb pain: evidence from two cases. Front Neurol 2018;9:67.

109. Trojan J, Diers M, Fuchs X, et al. An augmented reality home-training system based on the mirror training and imagery approach. Behav Res Methods 2014;46(3):634–40.

110. Johnson MI, Bjordal JM. Transcutaneous electrical nerve stimulation for the management of painful conditions: focus on neuropathic pain. Expert Rev Neurother 2011;11(5):735–53.

111. Bjordal JM, Johnson MI, Ljunggreen AE. Transcutaneous electrical nerve stimulation (TENS) can reduce postoperative analgesic consumption. A meta-analysis with assessment of optimal treatment parameters for postoperative pain. Eur J Pain 2003;7(2):181–8.

112. Sluka KA, Bjordal JM, Marchand S, et al. What makes transcutaneous electrical nerve stimulation work? Making sense of the mixed results in the clinical literature. Phys Ther 2013;93(10):1397–402.

113. Santos CM, Francischi JN, Lima-Paiva P, et al. Effect of transcutaneous electrical stimulation on nociception and edema induced by peripheral serotonin. Int J Neurosci 2013;123(7):507–15.

114. Melzack R, Wall PD. Pain mechanisms: a new theory. Science 1965;150(3699):971–9.

115. Wall PD, Sweet WH. Temporary abolition of pain in man. Science 1967;155(3758):108–9.

116. Gibson W, Wand BM, O'Connell NE. Transcutaneous electrical nerve stimulation (TENS) for neuropathic pain in adults. Cochrane Database Syst Rev 2017;9:CD011976.

117. Di Rollo A, Pallanti S. Phantom limb pain: low frequency repetitive transcranial magnetic stimulation in unaffected hemisphere. Case Rep Med 2011; 2011:130751.

118. Ahmed MA, Mohamed SA, Sayed D. Long-term antalgic effects of repetitive transcranial magnetic stimulation of motor cortex and serum beta-endorphin in patients with phantom pain. Neurol Res 2011;33(9):953–8.

119. Bolognini N, Olgiati E, Maravita A, et al. Motor and parietal cortex stimulation for phantom limb pain and sensations. Pain 2013;154(8):1274–80.

120. Bolognini N, Spandri V, Olgiati E, et al. Long-term analgesic effects of transcranial direct current stimulation of the motor cortex on phantom limb and stump pain: a case report. J Pain Symptom Manage 2013;46(4):e1–4.

121. Grammer GG, Williams-Joseph S, Cesar A, et al. Significant reduction in phantom limb pain after low-frequency repetitive transcranial magnetic stimulation to the primary sensory cortex. Mil Med 2015;180(1):e126–8.

122. Lee JH, Byun JH, Choe YR, et al. Successful treatment of phantom limb pain by 1 Hz repetitive transcranial magnetic stimulation over affected supplementary motor complex: a case report. Ann Rehabil Med 2015;39(4):630–3.

123. Malavera A, Silva FA, Fregni F, et al. Repetitive transcranial magnetic stimulation for phantom limb pain in land mine victims: a double-blinded, randomized, sham-controlled trial. J Pain 2016; 17(8):911–8.

Traditional Neuroma Management

Brian W. Starr, MD[a],*, Kevin C. Chung, MD, MS[b,1]

KEYWORDS

- Neuroma • Surgical management • Amputation • Nerve repair

KEY POINTS

- The experienced surgeon has more options than ever before in the prevention and management of problematic neuromas.
- At the time of known or suspected peripheral nerve injury: if the distal nerve segment is present, perform meticulous, tension-free repair; if the distal nerve segment is absent (ie, amputation), consider traction neurectomy versus transposition technique.
- When physical examination is consistent with painful neuroma formation: if the distal nerve segment is present (ie, neuroma in continuity), resect the neuroma and perform a technically sound, tension-free nerve repair with liberal use of nerve grafts; if the distal nerve segment is absent, resect the neuroma and transpose the regenerating nerve, giving it a new distal target protected from external stimuli.
- Consider targeted muscle reinnervation and regenerative peripheral nerve interface refractory cases and in younger, active patients with more proximal amputations.

INTRODUCTION

Treatment of the symptomatic, painful neuroma is a challenging problem with no clear consensus on optimal management. Review of existing literature reveals more than 150 various techniques and protocols for prevention, modulation, and treatment of neuroma pain.[1,2] All cut or damaged nerves form neuromas, but some form symptomatic, painful neuromas. Symptomatic neuromas are defined as neuromas that produce bothersome pain, cold intolerance, paresthesia, numbness, or electrical sensitivity.[1,3–6] Multiple studies have delineated that peripheral nerve injury and, more specifically, neuroma pain, can have profound detrimental effects on psychosocial well-being, limb function, and the ability to maintain gainful employment.[3,7,8] Traditional neuroma management consists of an array of surgical and nonsurgical interventions (as discussed in Kao and Liu's article, "Non-surgical Approaches to Neuroma Management," in this issue), including pharmacologic therapy, occupational therapy, and various desensitization techniques. Surgical management can be divided into primary management at the time of the initial peripheral nerve injury and secondary management, after a symptomatic neuroma has developed.

A critical distinction depends on whether neurorrhaphy can be performed at the time of the acute nerve injury (ie, primary management). If the regenerating nerve lacks an available distal target, as is the case in amputations, a neuroma invariably forms. At this point, the key questions become: (1) What can be done to minimize the risk of symptomatic neuroma formation? and (2) How to proceed once a symptomatic neuroma has

[a] Section of Plastic Surgery, University of Cincinnati Medical Center, 231 Albert Sabin Way, Mail Location: 0513, Cincinnati, OH 45229, USA; [b] Section of Plastic Surgery, The University of Michigan Health System, 1500 East Medical Center Drive, 2130 Taubman Center, SPC 5340, Ann Arbor, MI 48109-5340, USA
[1] Senior author
* Corresponding author.
E-mail address: starrbn@ucmail.uc.edu

Hand Clin 37 (2021) 335–344
https://doi.org/10.1016/j.hcl.2021.04.002

developed? With so many different techniques and approaches, this article aims to highlight the most common approaches for traditional neuroma management and the physiologic basis for their use.

ANATOMY AND PHYSIOLOGY OF NEUROMA

The impact that traumatic injury has on peripheral nerves is highly variable, depending on multiple patient and environmental factors, and is not limited to mechanism and severity of injury. Symptomatic neuromas can form as the result of chronic, repetitive trauma—as is the case with Morton neuroma and bowler thumb—or from acute nerve injury. The classically described Sunderland classification of nerve injuries describes the spectrum of neuronal trauma from neuropraxic (type I) to complete disruption and neurotmesis (type V).[9] In type I injuries, the extent of damage is contained to the insulating myelin sheath and its microenvironment, without affecting the inner axon. These injuries spontaneously recover through regeneration of myelin and restoration of the microenvironment.

In contrast to neuropraxic injuries, axonotometic injuries (types II–V) incite a cascade of events as a direct result of axonal discontinuity and separation of the cell body from the distal axon. Within 48 hours of axonotmesis, wallerian degeneration and the process of breaking down and eliminating inhibitory debris ensues. Myelinating Schwann cells distal to the injury dissociate from their myelin, release cytokines and growth factors, and proliferate. The nonfenestrated endothelial cells and tight junctions of the blood-nerve barrier become compromised and reach maximum permeability at 4 days to 7 days postinjury. Proliferating Schwann cells and activated macrophages phagocytize cellular debris and help to recruit new Schwann cells and to facilitate axon regeneration. Interdigitating Schwann cells form the basis for bands of Büngner and the subsequent sprouting of regenerating axons that make up the growth cone. The aligned basal lamina of the bands of Büngner form endoneurial tubes that secrete trophic factors and effectively guide the regenerating axon toward its distal target.[9–13]

If the regenerating nerve lacks a distal target or becomes impeded by scar, aberrant tissue, or debris, the sprouting axons deteriorate into a disorganized bundle of immature axons and connective tissue known as a neuroma.[11,12,14] Neuroma pain is multifactorial and can arise from a plethora of causes, including traction from scar tissue, compression by overlying soft tissue, ischemic changes, ectopic clusters of ion channels, central sensitization, and psychosocial factors.[15] Within the neuroma, sodium channels abnormally accumulate and lead to increased excitability that can present clinically as hypersensitivity and pain.[16,17] Acute inflammation and vasodilation lead to an influx of serotonin, bradykinin, histamine, and substance P. Nociceptors, including C and A delta nerve fibers, become sensitized by the local inflammatory response and subsequently up-regulate the transduction of painful impulses, while simultaneously lowering the threshold for transmission.[1,18] The chaotic arrangement of regenerating fascicles also may attempt to reinnervate the skin and superficial soft tissue, where they may be prone to hyperexcitability. Over time, constant stimulation of glial cells and subsequent cytokine release in the central nervous system fundamentally alter central neurophysiology and may contribute to chronic pain.[19]

The overwhelming majority of neuromas are asymptomatic. The incidence of symptomatic neuroma formation ranges from 4% to 25% for upper extremity amputations and 11% to 32% for lower extremity amputations.[4,20–25] van der Avoort and colleagues[22] reviewed 583 cases of hand trauma with peripheral nerve injury, of which 177 patients sustained digit amputations. In the amputation subset, where no neurorrhaphy could be performed, 7.8% of patients subsequently developed symptomatic neuromas.[22] Similarly, in a review of 1083 patients who underwent digital amputation, Eberlin and colleagues found 71 patients (6.6%) who developed painful neuromas. In this study, younger age, workers' compensation injuries, index finger injuries, and avulsion mechanisms were associated with statistically significant increases with symptomatic neuroma formation.[20]

SURGICAL TECHNIQUES
Primary Management (Prevention)

Distal nerve segment is present
A variety of surgical techniques have been reported in an attempt to prevent symptomatic neuroma formation. Management of the patient with a transected nerve and available distal nerve is fairly straightforward. The surgeon must perform a technically sound, tension-free nerve repair, utilizing nerve grafts for larger gaps as needed. Hollow tube–assisted repairs (conduit, connector, and so forth) can be used effectively in gaps up to 6 mm.[26,27] For larger gaps, nerve allografts have demonstrated favorable outcomes in several recent studies.[28,29] In experienced hands, with meticulous technique, symptomatic neuroma formation following primary nerve repair is rare. In

the previously cited report by van der Avoort and colleagues,[22] of 406 patients who sustained digital nerve injury and underwent neurorrhaphy, only 4 patients (1%) developed symptomatic neuromas.

Distal nerve segment is absent

Management of nerve stumps, when no distal nerve segment is available, as is the case in amputations, is a more challenging problem.[30–32] Traditional prevention strategies, prior to the development of targeted muscle reinnervation (TMR) and regenerative peripheral nerve interface (RPNI) surgery, often have not sought to prevent neuroma formation but rather to position the expected neuroma in a location where it is less prone to irritating forces that may exacerbate symptoms. Historically, traction neurectomy is the most common primary management technique used to prevent symptomatic neuroma pain.[33,34] This approach requires proximal dissection and skeletonization of the involved nerve. The terminal sensory nerve is placed on traction and sharply divided proximally, thus allowing the nerve end to retract away from the end of the healing limb or digit stump. Despite its prevalence, few studies have sought to directly compare traction neurectomy to other techniques in either primary or secondary neuroma management. Existing literature indicates, however, that traction neurectomy likely is less effective than more complex strategies, especially in more proximal amputations.[35,36] Economides and colleagues[36] retrospectively compared 17 patients who underwent transfemoral amputations and were treated with either traction neurectomy alone or nerve wrapping and peroneal-to-tibial nerve coaptation. At 6-month follow-up, the investigators found that the cohort treated with traction neurectomy alone was associated with higher visual analog scale (VAS) pain scores, phantom pain, and neuroma formation, with lower ambulation rates.[36] Pet and colleagues[35] raise similar questions regarding the effectiveness of traction neurectomy alone in secondary neuroma management. In a review of 38 patients with established, symptomatic lower extremity neuromas treated with traction neurectomy, Pet and colleagues reported that 42% failed to demonstrate sustained symptomatic improvement at 37-month follow-up. Despite its shortcomings, traction neurectomy frequently is implemented, especially in the digits, because it is quick and simple to perform. More recent innovations in preventing and treating symptomatic neuromas, including RPNI and TMR, are fundamentally different compared with traditional techniques discussed herein and are discussed in subsequent articles.

Secondary Management Diagnosis

As with any challenging clinical problem, the first step in effective treatment is to arrive at the correct diagnosis. A thorough history and physical examination are essential. The surgeon must distinguish between compression neuropathy and painful neuroma by elucidating details surrounding the timeline of symptoms, mechanism of injury, and exacerbating factors. Patients with symptomatic neuromas frequently present with pain, cold intolerance, paresthesia, numbness, or electrical sensitivity in the setting of acute or chronic trauma. A Tinel sign over the involved region is common but not a necessity.

Distal nerve segment is present

Surgical treatment of a symptomatic neuroma can be divided into 2 broad categories, depending on the availability of the distal nerve segment. In the setting of a neuroma-in-continuity (**Fig. 1**) or a neuroma where a distal nerve segment is present, surgical management typically requires resection of the neuroma and reconstruction of the nerve. Patient expectations and goals of treatment must be discussed carefully preoperatively, especially when a patient presents with a neuroma-in-continuity. The surgeon and patient must weigh carefully the implications of surgical intervention when mixed and motor nerves are involved. Following resection of a neuroma, the size of the nerve gap determines the need for an interposition autograft or allograft. In situations where the nerve gap is less than 6 mm, the nerve ends may be amenable to hollow tube–assisted repair (**Fig. 2**).[26,27] In most clinical scenarios, however, resection of the neuroma produces a larger nerve gap that precludes the use of this approach and instead requires interposition autografting or allografting (**Fig. 3**).[37] As alluded to previously, nerve allografts repeatedly have demonstrated their clinical utility. The predominant benefit of utilizing processed nerve allograft is the elimination of donor-site morbidity by allaying fears of a symptomatic neuroma forming at the site of would-be autograft harvest. In a retrospective review of 22 patients treated with interposition nerve allografts for symptomatic lower extremity neuromas, Souza and colleagues[38] demonstrated a significant reduction in pain scores documented at an average of 15-month follow-up.

Distal nerve segment is absent

A multitude of surgical approaches are used in the treatment of symptomatic neuromas that occur secondary to limb and digit amputations. The most common treatment method is resection of the neuroma and transposition of the proximal

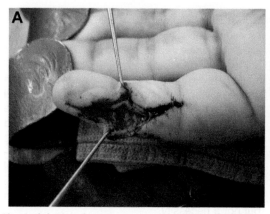
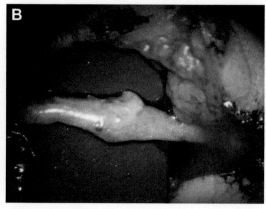

Fig. 1. (*A*) Digital nerve neuroma-in-continuity, (*B*) same image, magnified.

nerve stump into adjacent tissue that is less prone to mechanical stimulation.[1,33,37]

Transposition into Innervated Muscle

A 2018 comparative meta-analysis by Poppler and colleagues[39] demonstrated that excision and transposition is the most widespread strategy for secondary neuroma management (**Fig. 4**). In their review, 63% of studies used some variation of the excision and transposition approach.[39] Early reports of implantation of a sensory nerve into muscle in hopes of decreasing peripheral nerve pain and excitability date back to the early to mid-1900s.[40–42] Mackinnon[1] and Dellon popularized this concept for neuroma treatment in the 1980s.[43–46] In addition to reducing the nerve's exposure to noxious mechanical stimuli and preventing axon sprouting toward the skin, this technique also serves to potentiate the surrounding microenvironment, decreasing myofibroblast infiltration and neuroma size.[47–49] In a series of 78 neuromas treated with excision and transposition into nearby muscle, Dellon and Mackinnon[43] reported "good-to-excellent" results with an average follow-up of 31 months. In a separate study examining neuromas of the foot and ankle, Dellon and Aszmann[45] reported that excising the neuroma and transposing the nerve away from the joint, into adjacent muscle, produced "excellent" results at mean follow-up of 29 months.

Neurolysis and Coverage

Multiple investigators have reported effective use of vascularized local flaps for treatment of symptomatic neuromas.[50–54] In contrast to the excision and transposition technique, this approach can be applied more readily to challenging neuromas in continuity. The theoretic benefits of this technique include improving vascularity and facilitating nerve gliding, in addition to shielding the nerve from mechanical stimulation.[51] In their 1996 report, Rose and colleagues[54] demonstrated relief of digital neuroma symptoms in all patients treated with neurolysis and coverage with intrinsic muscle flaps. In this series, 4 patients were treated with lumbrical muscle flaps, 2 were treated with abductor muscle flaps, and 2 with adductor muscle flaps.[54] Similarly, Adani and colleagues[50] found that neuromas in continuity involving the median nerve at the wrist could be effectively managed

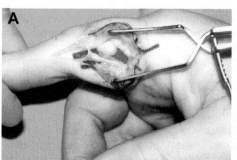
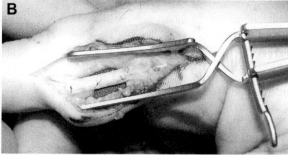

Fig. 2. (*A*) Digital nerve neuroma-in-continuity with branching to skin. (*B*) The neuroma-in-continuity has been treated with excision and reconstruction with a nerve conduit.

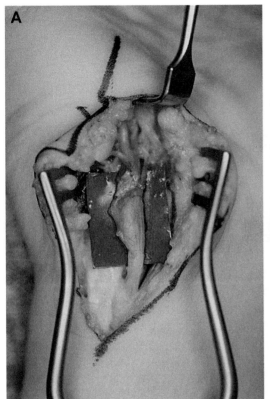 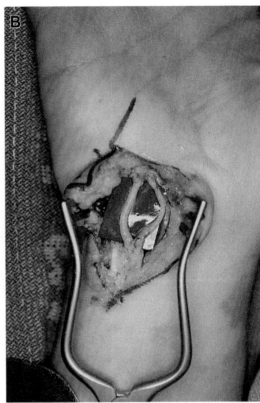

Fig. 3. (*A*) Ulnar nerve neuroma-in-continuity at the hypothenar eminence. (*B*) The neuroma-in-continuity has been treated with excision and reconstruction with sural nerve grafting.

with neurolysis and coverage with a pronator quadratus muscle flap. In their series of 9 patients, at mean 23-months' follow-up, 6 patients reported complete relief and 3 patients reported only mild, intermittent pain.[50] In an additional subset of patients treated with radial and ulnar artery adipofascial perforator flaps, Adani and colleagues[51] noted complete resolution of neuroma pain in 5 of 8 patients. In their comparative meta-analysis, Poppler and colleagues[39] found that in patients experiencing symptoms for over 2 years, 91% of patients noted improvement following treatment with neurolysis and coverage.

Transposition into Vein

Although implemented less routinely than excision and transposition into muscle, multiple investigators have demonstrated promising results with the excision and transposition into vein technique. This concept first was described in 1998 by Herbert and Filan,[55] who reported effective resolution of neuroma symptoms in 11 of 14 patients at a mean follow-up of 15 months. In this technique, the neuroma is resected and the proximal nerve stump is secured within the lumen of a nearby

vein in an end-to-end or end-to-side fashion. The theory behind this method is that the organized structure of the vein and its endothelial lining serve to reduce chaotic axonal sprouting. It also has been hypothesized that blood flow effectively clears neurotrophic factors that contribute to neuroma formation.[56–59] On histology, Herbert and Filan[55] demonstrated that following transposition into a vein, regenerating axons were more organized, with parallel fascicular architecture. In a well-designed, prospective, double-blind study comparing nerve transposition into muscle with transposition into vein, Balcin and colleagues[60] compared 20 patients with symptomatic lower extremity neuromas. At 12-month follow-up, transposition into vein significantly improved pain scores as measured on VAS and significantly improved function and level of activity.[60]

Transposition into Bone

Initially described by Boldrey in 1943,[61] intraosseous transposition as a technique for treatment of symptomatic neuromas gained in popularity in the 1980s. Multiple investigators reported success in independent, small series of patients treated

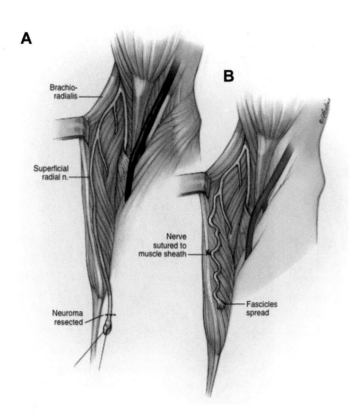

Fig. 4. (*A*) Diagram demonstrating neuroma resection (*B*) and transposition into adjacent muscle. n, nerve. (Copyright Elizabeth Martin - Green's Operative Hand Surgery 2010, Figure 32.26.)

with this technique.[62–64] In the largest series of patients treated with intraosseous transposition, Hazari and Elliot[65] retrospectively reviewed 104 painful nerves in 57 digits in 48 patients. They reported complete resolution of pain at the primary site in 98% of patients. Their specific approach consisted of dissecting the involved nerve proximally and transecting it prior to placing it in a bone tunnel in the proximal phalanx or metacarpal. The investigators note the importance of ensuring the nerve is not on tension and of beveling the bone tunnel edges in order to avoid compression points. This technique is most useful in clinical scenarios, such as digital neuromas, where additional soft tissue coverage is limited. In a 2016 review of surgical treatment of upper extremity pain, Dellon[66] states that implantation into bone remains a reasonable option for treatment of digital neuromas. In the authors' experience, this technique is useful in rare and refractory clinical scenarios. The morbidity associated with drilling bone tunnels should not be overlooked and the authors do not recommend this technique for routine use.

Centrocentral neurorrhaphy

The technique of centrocentral neurorrhaphy coapts 2, otherwise independent, adjacent nerves (ie, digital nerves) or coapts separate fascicles of the same nerve following intraneural dissection. This technique was introduced by Gorkisch and colleagues[67] in 1984 as a method for preventing digital neuroma formation following amputation. Histologic examination demonstrates reduction in fascicular escape with axons surrounded by intact perineurium and ultimately decreased the size of the end-neuroma.[68] In a randomized control trial studying patients who sustained digit amputations, Belcher and Pandya[32] compared 60 digits treated with either simple nerve transection or with centrocentral neurorrhaphy. The investigators of this study found no difference in resting pain, cold intolerance, or perceived tenderness between the 2 cohorts.[32] The authors discuss this technique primarily for historical context and for completeness. In the absence of established clinical benefit, the authors would not recommend its use in practice.

Nerve Capping

In 1976, Tupper and Booth[69] introduced the concept of excision and capping in an attempt to control immature sprouting axons and limit painful neuroma formation. Silicone caps have been shown to inhibit painful neuroma formation in part through the down-regulation of nerve growth factor and inflammatory markers.[70,71] This technique requires excision of the neuroma and placement of a silicone cap over the cut end. Swanson and colleagues[71] also reported promising results with this technique, noting resolution of neuroma symptoms in 24 of 26 patients at approximately 3-year follow-up. In a review of the surgical treatment of 348 symptomatic neuromas, Tupper reported that 65% of cases achieved "excellent or satisfactory" results with simple neuroma excision alone. In 32 cases that failed simple neurectomy alone, patients were treated with secondary excision and silicone capping. In long-term follow-up, however, Tupper and Booth[69] reported that there was no benefit of capping compared with simple excision alone. Although silicone caps long since have fallen out of favor, more recent literature has advocated for capping terminal nerve ends with other, more biocompatible materials, including vein and nerve allograft.[72–74] In a 2019 publication in the *Journal of Neurosurgery*, Onode and colleagues[73] report that the use of bioabsorbable nerve conduit caps effectively limits perineural inflammation, scar formation, and neuropathic pain, in a rat amputation model. Despite promising reports utilizing newer capping techniques, real-world clinical data are lacking and the authors, therefore, are unable to advocate for their routine use in practice.

SUMMARY

In the first prospective, randomized control trial comparing traditional transposition techniques to TMR, Dumanian and colleagues[75] found that the TMR cohort had measurable improvements in both phantom limb and neuroma pain at 1-year follow-up. Similarly, supportive evidence for RPNI continues to mount. Cederna and colleagues[76,77] repeatedly have demonstrated the effectiveness of RPNI in both treating and preventing symptomatic neuromas. With the development of newer techniques for symptomatic neuroma treatment, such as RPNI and TMR, transposition and coverage techniques often have been referred to as passive techniques. In spite of its negative connotation, traditional passive techniques remain reasonable modalities and yield positive results in a majority of patients treated. In arguably the most thorough review of traditional neuroma management techniques, Poppler and colleagues[39] report a "meaningful reduction in pain" in 77% of patients treated by any means, despite not being able to find a statistically significant difference between specific operative techniques. Although additional well-designed, comparative studies examining outcomes and cost are needed, the experienced surgeon has more options than ever before for the prevention and management of problematic neuromas. Critical appraisal of the existing literature reveals no single best treatment. Instead, surgeons have a plethora of useful techniques that can be implemented on a case-by-case basis to optimize outcomes. In the authors' practice, patients are screened and counseled carefully prior to any surgical undertaking. Despite its shortcomings, traction neurectomy remains the authors' first-line approach to primary management (prevention) in digital amputations. Similarly, in regard to secondary management, most patients achieve substantial symptomatic improvement with traditional transposition techniques. In refractory cases and in younger, active patients with more proximal amputations, the authors have a lower threshold for more complex approaches, including TMR and RPNI.

CLINICS CARE POINTS

- At the time of nerve injury, counsel patients regarding the risk of painful neuroma formation and take steps to reduce this risk.
- Use atraumatic technique and perform meticulous, tension-free nerve repairs.
- Perform traction neurectomy or a variation of nerve transposition at the time of primary amputation. If a symptomatic neuroma develops, excise the neuroma, and transpose the regenerating nerve, giving it a new distal target, protected from external stimuli.
- Consider TMR and RPNI in refractory cases and in younger, active patients with more proximal amputations.

DISCLOSURE

Dr K.C. Chung receives funding from the National Institutes of Health and book royalties from Wolters Kluwer and Elsevier. He is a consultant for Axogen.

REFERENCES

1. Mackinnon SE. Evaluation and treatment of the painful neuroma. Tech Hand Up Extrem Surg 1997;1(3): 195–212.
2. Guse DM, Moran SL. Outcomes of the surgical treatment of peripheral neuromas of the hand and forearm: a 25-year comparative outcome study. Ann Plast Surg 2013;71(6):654–8.

3. Domeshek LF, Krauss EM, Snyder-Warwick AK, et al. Surgical treatment of neuromas improves patient-reported pain, depression, and quality of life. Plast Reconstr Surg 2017;139(2):407–18.

4. Geraghty TJ, Jones LE. Painful neuromata following upper limb amputation. Prosthet Orthot Int 1996; 20(3):176–81.

5. Stokvis A, Ruijs AC, van Neck JW, et al. Cold intolerance in surgically treated neuroma patients: a prospective follow-up study. J Hand Surg Am 2009; 34(9):1689–95.

6. Stahl S, Rosenberg N. Surgical treatment of painful neuroma in medial antebrachial cutaneous nerve. Ann Plast Surg 2002;48(2):154–60.

7. Wojtkiewicz DM, Saunders J, Domeshek L, et al. Social impact of peripheral nerve injuries. Hand (N Y) 2015;10(2):161–7.

8. Novak CB, van Vliet D, Mackinnon SE. Subjective outcome following surgical management of upper extremity neuromas. J Hand Surg Am 1995;20(2): 221–6.

9. Sunderland S. The anatomy and physiology of nerve injury. Muscle Nerve 1990;13(9):771–84.

10. Gaudet AD, Popovich PG, Ramer MS. Wallerian degeneration: gaining perspective on inflammatory events after peripheral nerve injury. J Neuroinflammation 2011;8:110.

11. Lee SK, Wolfe SW. Peripheral nerve injury and repair. J Am Acad Orthop Surg 2000;8(4):243–52.

12. Flores AJ, Lavernia CJ, Owens PW. Anatomy and physiology of peripheral nerve injury and repair. Am J Orthop 2000;29(3):167–73.

13. Navarro X, Vivó M, Valero-Cabré A. Neural plasticity after peripheral nerve injury and regeneration. Prog Neurobiol 2007;82(4):163–201.

14. Fried K, Govrin-Lippmann R, Rosenthal F, et al. Ultrastructure of afferent axon endings in a neuroma. J Neurocytol 1991;20(8):682–701.

15. Rajput K, Reddy S, Shankar H. Painful neuromas. Clin J Pain 2012;28(7):639–45.

16. England JD, Happel LT, Kline DG, et al. Sodium channel accumulation in humans with painful neuromas. Neurology 1996;47(1):272–6.

17. Devor M. Sodium channels and mechanisms of neuropathic pain. J Pain 2006;7(1 Suppl 1):S3–12.

18. Dahl JB, Mathiesen O, Møiniche S. Protective pre-medication': an option with gabapentin and related drugs? A review of gabapentin and pregabalin in in the treatment of post-operative pain. Acta Anaesthesiol Scand 2004;48(9):1130–6.

19. Pruimboom L, van Dam AC. Chronic pain: a non-use disease. Med Hypotheses 2007;68(3):506–11.

20. Vlot MA, Wilkens SC, Chen NC, et al. Symptomatic neuroma following initial amputation for traumatic digital amputation. J Hand Surg Am 2018;43(1):86.e1-e8.

21. Fisher GT, Boswick JA Jr. Neuroma formation following digital amputations. J Trauma 1983;23(2): 136–42.

22. van der Avoort DJ, Hovius SE, Selles RW, et al. The incidence of symptomatic neuroma in amputation and neurorrhaphy patients. J Plast Reconstr Aesthet Surg 2013;66(10):1330–4.

23. Ebrahimzadeh MH, Fattahi AS. Long-term clinical outcomes of iranian veterans with unilateral transfemoral amputation. Disabil Rehabil 2009;31(22):1873–7.

24. Ebrahimzadeh MH, Hariri S. Long-term outcomes of unilateral transtibial amputations. Mil Med 2009; 174(6):593–7.

25. Tintle SM, Shawen SB, Forsberg JA, et al. Reoperation after combat-related major lower extremity amputations. J Orthop Trauma 2014;28(4):232–7.

26. Moore AM, Kasukurthi R, Magill CK, et al. Limitations of conduits in peripheral nerve repairs. Hand (N Y) 2009;4(2):180–6.

27. Boeckstyns ME, Sørensen AI, Viñeta JF, et al. Collagen conduit versus microsurgical neurorrhaphy: 2-year follow-up of a prospective, blinded clinical and electro-physiological multicenter randomized, controlled trial. J Hand Surg Am 2013;38(12):2405–11.

28. Tang P, Whiteman DR, Voigt C, et al. No difference in outcomes detected between decellular nerve allograft and cable autograft in rat sciatic nerve defects. J Bone Joint Surg Am 2019;101(10):e42.

29. Mauch JT, Bae A, Shubinets V, et al. A systematic review of sensory outcomes of digital nerve gap reconstruction with autograft, allograft, and conduit. Ann Plast Surg 2019;82(4):S247–55.

30. Crosio A, Albo E, Marcoccio I, et al. Prevention of symptomatic neuroma in traumatic digital amputation: a RAND/UCLA appropriateness method consensus study. Injury 2020;51(Suppl 4):S103–7.

31. St-Laurent JY, Duclos L. Prevention of neuroma in elective digital amputations by utilization of neuro-vascular island flap. Ann Chir Main Memb Super 1996;15(1):50–4.

32. Belcher HJ, Pandya AN. Centro-central union for the prevention of neuroma formation after finger amputation. J Hand Surg Br 2000;25(2):154–9.

33. Ducic I, Mesbahi AN, Attinger CE, et al. The role of peripheral nerve surgery in the treatment of chronic pain associated with amputation stumps. Plast Reconstr Surg 2008;121(3):908–14.

34. Whipple RR, Unsell RS. Treatment of painful neuromas. Orthop Clin North Am 1988;19(1):175–85.

35. Pet MA, Ko JH, Friedly JL, et al. Traction neurectomy for treatment of painful residual limb neuroma in lower extremity amputees. J Orthop Trauma 2015;29(9):321.

36. Economides JM, DeFazio MV, Attinger CE, et al. Prevention of painful neuroma and phantom limb pain after transfemoral amputations through concomitant nerve coaptation and collagen nerve wrapping. Neurosurgery 2016;79(3):508–13.

37. Eberlin KR, Ducic I. Surgical algorithm for neuroma management: a changing treatment paradigm. Plast Reconstr Surg Glob Open 2018;6(10):e1952.

38. Souza JM, Purnell CA, Cheesborough JE, et al. Treatment of foot and ankle neuroma pain with processed nerve allografts. Foot Ankle Int 2016; 37(10):1098–105.

39. Poppler LH, Parikh RP, Bichanich MJ, et al. Surgical interventions for the treatment of painful neuroma: a comparative meta-analysis. Pain 2018;159(2):214–23.

40. Teneff S. Prevention of amputation neuroma. J Int Coll Surg 1949;12(1):16–20.

41. Moszkowicz L. Zur behandlung der schmerzhaften neurome. Zentrablbl Chir 1918;(45):547.

42. Munro D, Mallory GK. Elimination of the so-called amputation neuromas of divided peripheral nerves. N Engl J Med 1959;260(8):358–61.

43. Dellon AL, Mackinnon SE. Treatment of the painful neuroma by neuroma resection and muscle implantation. Plast Reconstr Surg 1986;77(3):427–38.

44. Evans GR, Dellon AL. Implantation of the palmar cutaneous branch of the median nerve into the pronator quadratus for treatment of painful neuroma. J Hand Surg Am 1994;19(2):203–6.

45. Dellon AL, Aszmann OC. Treatment of superficial and deep peroneal neuromas by resection and translocation of the nerves into the anterolateral compartment. Foot Ankle Int 1998;19(5):300–3.

46. Dellon AL, Mackinnon SE, Pestronk A. Implantation of sensory nerve into muscle: preliminary clinical and experimental observations on neuroma formation. Ann Plast Surg 1984;12(1):30–40.

47. Krishnan KG, Pinzer T, Schackert G. Coverage of painful peripheral nerve neuromas with vascularized soft tissue: method and results. Neurosurgery 2005; 56(2 Suppl):369–78.

48. Yan H, Gao W, Pan Z, et al. The expression of α-SMA in the painful traumatic neuroma: potential role in the pathobiology of neuropathic pain. J Neurotrauma 2012;29(18):2791–7.

49. Mackinnon SE, Dellon AL, Hudson AR, et al. Alteration of neuroma formation by manipulation of its microenvironment. Plast Reconstr Surg 1985;76(3): 345–53.

50. Adani R, Tarallo L, Battiston B, et al. Management of neuromas in continuity of the median nerve with the pronator quadratus muscle flap. Ann Plast Surg 2002;48(1):35–40.

51. Adani R, Tos P, Tarallo L, et al. Treatment of painful median nerve neuromas with radial and ulnar artery perforator adipofascial flaps. J Hand Surg Am 2014; 39(4):721–7.

52. Elliot D, Lloyd M, Hazari A, et al. Relief of the pain of neuromas-in-continuity and scarred median and ulnar nerves in the distal forearm and wrist by neurolysis, wrapping in vascularized forearm fascial flaps and adjunctive procedures. J Hand Surg Eur Vol 2010;35(7):575–82.

53. Kakinoki R, Ikeguchi R, Atiyya AN, et al. Treatment of posttraumatic painful neuromas at the digit tip using neurovascular island flaps. J Hand Surg Am 2008; 33(3):348–52.

54. Rose J, Belsky MR, Millender LH, et al. Intrinsic muscle flaps: the treatment of painful neuromas in continuity. J Hand Surg Am 1996;21(4):671–4.

55. Herbert TJ, Filan SL. Vein implantation for treatment of painful cutaneous neuromas. A preliminary report. J Hand Surg Br 1998;23(2):220–4.

56. Low CK, Chew SH, Song IC, et al. Implantation of a nerve ending into a vein. Clin Orthop Relat Res 2000;(379):242–6.

57. Koch H, Haas F, Hubmer M, et al. Treatment of painful neuroma by resection and nerve stump transplantation into a vein. Ann Plast Surg 2003;51(1):45–50.

58. Koch H, Herbert TJ, Kleinert R, et al. Influence of nerve stump transplantation into a vein on neuroma formation. Ann Plast Surg 2003;50(4):354–60.

59. Kakinoki R, Ikeguchi R, Matsumoto T, et al. Treatment of painful peripheral neuromas by vein implantation. Int Orthop 2003;27(1):60–4.

60. Balcin H, Erba P, Wettstein R, et al. A comparative study of two methods of surgical treatment for painful neuroma. J Bone Joint Surg Br 2009;91(6):803–8.

61. Boldrey E. Amputation neuroma in nerves implanted in bone. Ann Surg 1943;118(6):1052–7.

62. Mass DP, Ciano MC, Tortosa R, et al. Treatment of painful hand neuromas by their transfer into bone. Plast Reconstr Surg 1984;74(2):182–5.

63. Goldstein SA, Sturim HS. Intraosseous nerve transposition for treatment of painful neuromas. J Hand Surg Am 1985;10(2):270–4.

64. Hemmy DC. Intramedullary nerve implantation in amputation and other traumatic neuromas. J Neurosurg 1981;54(6):842–3.

65. Hazari A, Elliot D. Treatment of end-neuromas, neuromas-in-continuity and scarred nerves of the digits by proximal relocation. J Hand Surg Br 2004;29(4): 338–50.

66. Dellon AL. Surgical treatment of upper extremity pain. Hand Clin 2016;32(1):71–80.

67. Gorkisch K, Boese-Landgraf J, Vaubel E. Treatment and prevention of amputation neuromas in hand surgery. Plast Reconstr Surg 1984;73(2):293–9.

68. González-Darder J, Barberá J, Abellán MJ, et al. Centrocentral anastomosis in the prevention and treatment of painful terminal neuroma. an experimental study in the rat. J Neurosurg 1985;63(5):754–8.

69. Tupper JW, Booth DM. Treatment of painful neuromas of sensory nerves in the hand: a comparison of traditional and newer methods. J Hand Surg Am 1976;1(2):144–51.

70. Okuda T, Ishida O, Fujimoto Y, et al. The autotomy relief effect of a silicone tube covering the proximal nerve stump. J Orthop Res 2006;24(7):1427–37.

71. Swanson AB, Boeve NR, Lumsden RM. The prevention and treatment of amputation neuromata by silicone capping. J Hand Surg Am 1977;2(1):70–8.

72. Yan H, Zhang F, Kolkin J, et al. Mechanisms of nerve capping technique in prevention of painful neuroma formation. PLoS One 2014;9(4):e93973.

73. Onode E, Uemura T, Takamatsu K, et al. Nerve capping with a nerve conduit for the treatment of painful neuroma in the rat sciatic nerve. J Neurosurg 2019;132(3):856–64.

74. Galeano M, Manasseri B, Risitano G, et al. A free vein graft cap influences neuroma formation after nerve transection. Microsurgery 2009;29(7):568–72.

75. Dumanian GA, Potter BK, Mioton LM, et al. Targeted muscle reinnervation treats neuroma and phantom pain in major limb amputees: a randomized clinical trial. Ann Surg 2019;270(2):238–46.

76. Kubiak CA, Kemp SWP, Cederna PS, et al. Prophylactic regenerative peripheral nerve interfaces to prevent postamputation pain. Plast Reconstr Surg 2019;144(3):421e–30e.

77. Hooper RC, Cederna PS, Brown DL, et al. Regenerative peripheral nerve interfaces for the management of symptomatic hand and digital neuromas. Plast Reconstr Surg Glob Open 2020; 8(6):e2792.

Targeted Muscle Reinnervation for the Treatment of Neuroma

Lindsay E. Janes, MD, Megan E. Fracol, MD, Gregory A. Dumanian, MD,
Jason H. Ko, MD, MBA*

KEYWORDS

• Neuroma • Targeted muscle reinnervation • Nerve transfer • Neuropathic pain

KEY POINTS

- Targeted muscle reinnervation (TMR) was initially established to improve prosthetic function in upper-extremity amputees and has subsequently been proven to be effective in treating and preventing residual limb pain and phantom limb pain.
- Application of TMR has now extended beyond the amputee population to treat chronic neuroma pain in nonamputee patients whereby neuroma excision and nerve reconstruction are either not possible or have failed.
- Specific nerve transfer patterns have been described for performing TMR at the various upper- and lower-extremity amputation levels, although the exact pattern of nerve transfers is flexible and frequently adjusted dependent on patient anatomy and neuroma location.

INTRODUCTION

Neuromas form in response to peripheral nerve injury as the body's attempt at axonal regeneration becomes a mass of disorganized nerve endings and scar tissue. Neuromas may be irritated by light touch, pressure, and extremes in temperature, causing chronic intense localized and/or radiating pain. Although the symptoms of chronic neuroma pain are universally debilitating, the cause of the pain has a wide range, including neuroma-in-continuity from long-standing nerve compression, surgery or trauma, and end neuromas after neurotomy. Unfortunately, because of the lack of definitive treatments, opioids remain the cornerstone of neuroma pain management despite mixed efficacy and known risks.[1–3]

Targeted muscle reinnervation (TMR) is a nerve transfer procedure designed to reroute amputated nerve ends to nearby motor nerve branches, therein providing a physiologic healing mechanism for the amputated nerve end. Originally developed to provide intuitive myoelectric prosthesis control in upper-extremity amputees, TMR has been used to successfully *treat* chronic neuroma pain in both the amputee[4,5] and the nonamputee populations.[6,7] Further study has shown that TMR can *prevent* the development of chronic neuroma pain if performed at the time of amputation.[8,9]

Here, the authors provide an overview of TMR for the treatment of neuromas, focusing on patient evaluation, their surgical approach to neuroma treatment, and TMR techniques to treat neuromas in both the amputee and the nonamputee populations.

PREVALENCE/INCIDENCE

As many as 90% of amputees suffer from postamputation pain in the form of either local residual limb pain or phantom limb pain.[10,11] Neuromas, a specific cause of residual limb pain in amputees, have been reported to affect 25% to 71% of

Division of Plastic and Reconstructive Surgery, Department of Orthopaedic Surgery, Northwestern University Feinberg School of Medicine, 675 North St. Clair Street, Suite 19-250, Chicago, IL 60611, USA
* Corresponding author.
E-mail address: Jason.ko@nm.org

Hand Clin 37 (2021) 345–359
https://doi.org/10.1016/j.hcl.2021.05.002
0749-0712/21/© 2021 Elsevier Inc. All rights reserved.

amputees.[12,13] Approximately 31% to 34% of patients who undergo a lower-extremity amputation will not return to work[14,15]; 62% of those patients cite prosthesis-related problems as the cause.[14] For many patients, the inability to use a prosthesis is secondary to residual limb and phantom limb pain.[16–18] Furthermore, many patients report that their prosthesis worsens phantom limb pain, causing them to wear it for significantly fewer hours per day.[16] Postamputation pain can profoundly affect prosthetic fit and function, mobility, return to work and social activities, and overall quality of life.[19,20]

A recent large-scale cross-sectional survey of upper- and lower-extremity amputees across North America identified female sex, lower educational status, and trauma-related amputations as factors associated with higher odds of residual limb pain (Mioton and colleagues, submitted for publication). Neuromas are a significant contributor to chronic pain in the amputee and in turn can impact prosthesis wear, amputee functionality, and, ultimately, quality of life.[21]

Chronic pain, with neuromas being a significant contributor, affects 10% to 85% of postsurgical patients.[22,23] In hand surgery, specific operations are associated with inherent risks of local neuroma formation. For instance, after cubital tunnel release, neuromas of the medial antebrachial cutaneous (MABC) nerve have been reported to be as high as 30% and are a frequent cause for reoperation.[24] Similarly, neuromas of the palmar cutaneous branch of the median nerve used to be one of the most common complications after carpal tunnel release but can be avoided with appropriate incision placement.[25] The superficial branch of the radial nerve has been identified as particularly prone to neuroma formation because of tethering as it exits from the brachioradialis.[26] Thus, adequate knowledge of local nerves susceptible to injury for any given surgical approach can prevent long-term chronic pain and disability postoperatively. Similarly, this knowledge can aid in identification of neuromas postoperatively and facilitate appropriate treatment.

CURRENT EVIDENCE

Early studies demonstrated the efficacy of TMR for intuitive prosthetic control in upper-extremity amputees.[27,28] Animal and human data subsequently demonstrated the physiologic reinnervation of target muscles.[29,30] After continued observation of pain improvements in patients who underwent TMR for prosthesis control,[4] the first surgical randomized controlled trial for chronic neuroma-related residual limb pain and

phantom limb pain was initiated. In this trial, TMR resulted in improved phantom limb pain and trended toward improved residual limb pain in major limb amputees compared with standard therapy for neuroma excision and burying in a nearby muscle.[5] Given that neuroma-related residual limb pain is a frequent cause of reoperation[19] and that centralized, chronic pain is difficult to treat, TMR at the time of major limb amputation was introduced for preemptive management of residual limb and phantom limb pain.[8,19] In a multicenter cohort study of patients who underwent TMR at the time of major limb amputation, TMR patients reported significantly less residual limb and phantom limb pain compared with a cross-sectional control amputee cohort.[9] Further studies are needed to demonstrate the effect of TMR on functional outcomes, such as mobility and return to work.

PATIENT SELECTION

One of the most important factors leading to successful treatment of neuroma pain is a motivated patient with appropriate expectations from surgery. It is important to counsel patients that the postoperative pain course is variable. There is a spectrum of outcomes ranging from immediate pain relief upon arousal from anesthesia, months-long delay in pain relief, temporary increase in phantom limb pain, intermittent periods of pain relief followed by return of pain, or no change in pain. In the authors' experience, younger patients, with shorter periods between nerve injury and TMR, have the greatest success.

EVALUATION

Preoperative work up of the patient presenting with focal pain should begin with a detailed history: eliciting the onset of pain, duration of symptoms, exacerbating factors, prior surgery in the region, narcotic use, and prior treatments (surgical and/or medical). Examination should focus on the location of prior surgical scars, the location of Tinel sign or signs, dermatomal distributions of numbness, and the soft tissue envelope in amputee residual limbs.

Often, the combination of a dermatomal distribution of numbness and a focal Tinel sign in a region that correlates with the nerve supplying that dermatome is enough to diagnose a neuroma. However, in cases whereby it is uncertain or when patients present with more diffuse pain symptoms that could be attributable to neuromas in multiple locations, administration of 1 to 2 cc of local anesthetic in the region of the suspected neuroma or neuromas can be a quick diagnostic test performed in the clinic. The authors suggest patients wait about 30 minutes after local anesthetic injection to confirm the diagnostic accuracy of the test. If, after these 30 minutes, they report improvement in their symptoms, then it is a good sign that their symptoms are attributable to a specific neuroma. In still uncertain cases, ultrasound can be performed to confirm a neuroma or to distinguish between 2 adjacent peripheral nerves that could have neuromatous change (ie, superficial peroneal vs lateral sural nerves). As painful nerves identified in the operating room can have normal contour but are abnormal only by color and palpation, results from ultrasound are only moderately helpful at best for what is essentially a clinical diagnosis.

APPROACH

TMR is 1 of 3 procedures in the authors' treatment algorithm for neuromas. The authors prefer to reconstruct short nerve gaps (<3 cm) with nerve allograft.[31,32] If this fails, or in instances with nerve defects between 3 and 6 cm, the authors rarely will use the motor nerve to the vastus lateralis as nerve graft in order to avoid damage to an alternate sensory nerve and potential for sensory neuromas at the donor site. If this fails, or in nerve gaps larger than 6 cm that are deemed un-reconstructable, the authors will opt for TMR. They more and more often suspect that the quality of pain relief is better with TMR than with nerve allografts, and so their use of allografts has slightly gone down with time. Perhaps this is due to greater length of nerve resection with TMR as opposed to allografts, where there is a concomitant attempt to keep the allograft nerve length short. In the residual limb of amputees, TMR is also the authors' initial treatment for neuromas, given these are un-reconstructable (nowhere for the nerve end to go).

SURGICAL TECHNIQUES
Shoulder Disarticulation Amputee

TMR in the shoulder disarticulation amputee is performed for the major nerve branches of the brachial plexus: median, ulnar, radial, and musculocutaneous nerves (**Table 1**).[33] It is particularly important in these patients to assess for potential donor motor nerves as part of the preoperative work up, given that the nature of these injuries can be associated with more proximal or panbrachial plexus injuries. The pectoralis major is the primary motor target at the shoulder amputation level and can be assessed by asking the patient to flex the pectoralis or simulate pushing

their hands together. The latissimus dorsi is another common target that can be assessed by asking the patient to simulate adducting the arm or coughing.

In the operating room, the patient is positioned supine. A 6- to 8-cm incision is made 1 to 2 fingerbreadths inferior and parallel to the clavicle, starting at the level of the acromion and proceeding medially. When designing incision placement, the presence or absence of the humeral head should also be considered. In the absence of the humeral head (a true shoulder disarticulation), the muscles of the shoulder girdle will retract medially, and as such, the incision should be placed slightly more medial.

Dissection proceeds through subcutaneous tissues to the level of the pectoralis major. A stripe of fat will indicate the plane between the sternal and clavicular heads of the pectoralis, through which blunt dissection can be performed.

The pectoralis minor can be released for enhanced visualization. The lateral pectoral motor nerve branches to clavicular head of the pectoralis major, and the medial pectoral nerve branches are more inferior. Motor nerves are confirmed with a nerve stimulator. Last, the lateral chest wall is explored; the lateral edge of the latissimus dorsi is elevated, and the thoracodorsal nerve is identified coursing just inside this edge of the muscle. Now that all donor and recipient nerves have been identified, additional dissection is performed to gain appropriate length on donor and recipient nerve endings to allow tension-free coaptation. Although the exact pattern of nerve transfers is surgeon-dependent, the authors have found the following pattern tends to work well: musculocutaneous nerve to motor branch to clavicular head of pectoralis major (elbow flexion signal is most important for pattern recognition), median nerve to upper portion of sternal head of pectoralis, ulnar nerve to lower portion of sternal head of pectoralis, and radial nerve to thoracodorsal nerve (**Figs. 1 and 2**).[8,33]

Transhumeral Amputee

In the transhumeral amputee, 3 major nerves are considered for TMR: the median, the ulnar, and the radial nerves (**Table 2**).

Transhumeral TMR can be performed acutely through the amputation site (**Fig. 3**) or in delayed fashion classically through a 2-incision approach (**Fig. 4**), although recently described through a single anterior incision.[34] It is important to ask the patient to actively flex their biceps and triceps muscle bellies in the preoperative holding area to help with orientation. The raphe between the 2

Table 1
Example pattern of targeted muscle reinnervation nerve transfers in a shoulder disarticulation amputee

Donor Nerve	Recipient Nerve	Muscle Innervated	Special Considerations
Musculocutaneous	Pectoral	Clavicular head of pectoralis major	These amputees often have extensive polytrauma, which can limit the number of donor targets and the soft tissue envelope. Evaluate for proximal brachial plexus injury before TMR
Median	Pectoral	Upper sternal head of pectoralis major	
Ulnar	Pectoral	Lower sternal head of pectoralis major	
Radial	Thoracodorsal	Latissimus	

heads of the biceps and between heads of the triceps is marked for incision placement. Typically, the patient can be positioned supine for the anterior TMR and then repositioned prone for the posterior TMR, or the patient can be placed in the lateral decubitus position to avoid position changes intraoperatively. Anteriorly, the incision between the 2 heads of the biceps is made. Exposing this interval will reveal the course of the musculocutaneous nerve, giving off branches to the biceps first, followed distally by branches to the brachialis (if sufficient arm length remains) and the final distal continuation of the nerve as the lateral antebrachial cutaneous (LABC). The branch to the short head of the biceps and the branch to the brachialis are tagged with vessel loops, leaving the branch to the long head of the biceps intact to maintain the elbow flexion signal. Next, the median nerve is located, coursing next

to the brachial artery. The ulnar nerve can then be identified just medial to the median nerve and deep to the MABC nerve. The median and ulnar nerves are transected distally and dissected proximally for length. These nerves are then transposed under the short head of the biceps to bring them into the interval between the heads of the biceps. Again, the exact pattern of nerve transfers is flexible, but the authors have found that transferring the median nerve to the motor branch to the short head of the biceps and the ulnar nerve to the motor nerve to the brachialis works well.

Once the anterior side is complete, the posterior arm is exposed for the radial nerve TMR (**Fig. 5**). The incision is made between the long and lateral heads of the triceps. The radial nerve is identified in this interspace. It is transected distally (again through healthy fascicles, just proximal to neuroma) and dissected proximally. The most distal

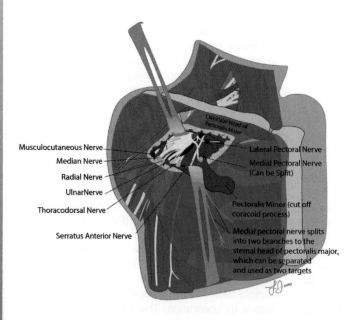

Fig. 1. Approach to TMR for shoulder disarticulation amputees. Musculocutaneous nerve to motor branch to clavicular head of pectoralis major (*purple dots*), median nerve to upper portion of sternal head of pectoralis (*green dots*), ulnar nerve to lower portion of sternal head of pectoralis (*pink dots*), and radial nerve to thoracodorsal nerve (*blue dots*).

Musculocutaneous Nerve
Median Nerve
Radial Nerve
UlnarNerve
Thoracodorsal Nerve
Serratus Anterior Nerve

Clavicular Head of Pectoralis Major
Lateral Pectoral Nerve
Medial Pectoral Nerve (Can be Split)
Pectoralis Minor (cut off coracoid process)
Medial pectoral nerve splits into two branches to the sternal head of pectoralis major, which can be separated and used as two targets

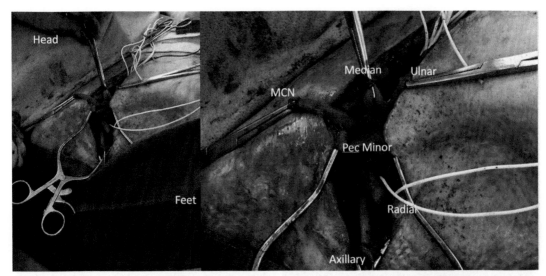

Fig. 2. TMR for shoulder disarticulation amputee. MCN, musculocutaneous nerve; Pec, pectoralis.

motor branch is to the lateral head and is thus the ideal target for TMR, thereby preserving more proximal radial nerve innervation to the medial and long heads. The motor branch to the lateral head is cut proximally, and the radial nerve proper is coapted to this motor branch.

Transradial Amputee

TMR in the transradial amputee is primarily focused on the median and ulnar nerves, as most of the radial nerve-innervated structures will remain in the residual limb (**Table 3**). Sensory nerves that can be considered for inclusion are the superficial branch of the radial nerve, the MABC, and the LABC.

Transradial TMR can be performed acutely through the amputation site or in delayed fashion via a 1- or 2-incision approach.[35] For a single-incision approach, the incision is designed about

10 cm distal to the antecubital fossa and then curved toward the ulnar nerve proximally (as demonstrated in **Figs. 6** and **7**). For a 2-incision approach, the first incision is just distal to the antecubital fossa and just medial to the insertion of the biceps tendon (the same approach used for a pronator syndrome release). This approach will expose the median nerve as it courses under the pronator quadratus and fibrous arch of the flexor digitorum superficialis (FDS). The median nerve is transected distally and coapted to motor nerves to the FDS or flexor digitorum profundus (FDP), or alternatively can be coapted to the anterior interosseous nerve (AIN) itself. The second incision is a very distally placed cubital tunnel incision (extending several centimeters distal to the medial epicondyle). The ulnar nerve is identified as it courses between the 2 heads of the flexor carpi ulnaris (FCU) and is coapted to a motor nerve to the FCU. These motor nerves

Table 2
Example pattern of targeted muscle reinnervation nerve transfers in a transhumeral amputee

Donor Nerve	Recipient Nerve	Muscle Innervated	Special Considerations
Median	Musculocutaneous motor branch	Short head of biceps	When performing in a delayed fashion, be sure to mark the raphe between the biceps muscle bellies and between the triceps muscle bellies with the patient actively firing, otherwise the lack of landmarks can be disorienting and complicate incision placement
Ulnar	Musculocutaneous motor branch	Brachialis	
Radial	Radial motor branch	Lateral head of triceps	

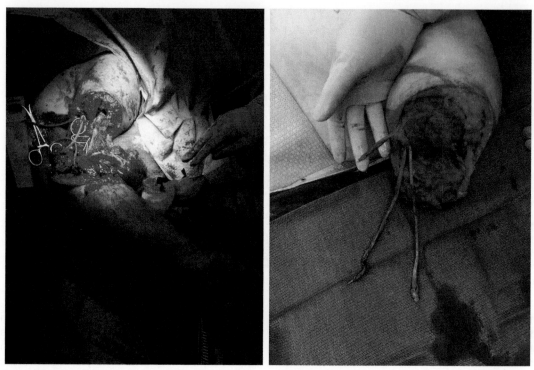

Fig. 3. The approach to performing TMR acutely at the time of transhumeral amputation through the amputation site.

to the FCU are relatively proximally located in proportion to the length of the muscle belly. If the superficial branch of the radial nerve, MABC, or LABC requires neuroma treatment, incisions can be designed over the Tinel sign and motor nerves to the FDS or FDP muscles identified for coaptation. For proximal amputations, a motor branch coursing into the brachioradialis can be identified above the elbow flexion crease on the medial surface of the muscle and adjacent to the radial nerve itself. In long transradial amputations, the pronator quadratus motor nerve can accept the distal radial nerve or the LABC. As there are no currently marketed prosthetics for transradial amputations that use TMR, all these nerve transfer procedures are only for pain control and not for signal acquisition. When these prosthetics become available, the superficial-most muscles of the brachioradialis and the FCU will be the best targets.

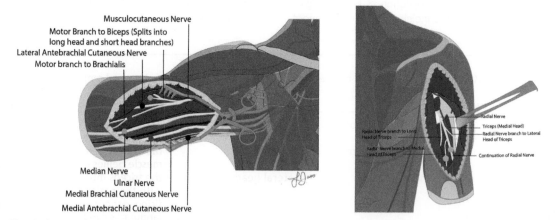

Fig. 4. Approach to TMR for transhumeral amputees. Median nerve to motor branch to short head of biceps (*green dots*), ulnar nerve to motor branch to brachialis (*pink dots*), radial nerve to motor branch to triceps (*blue dots*). LABC and MABC (*black dots*) can be buried in muscle because of lack of available motor targets.

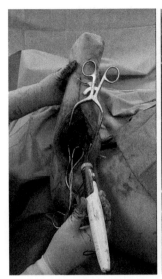 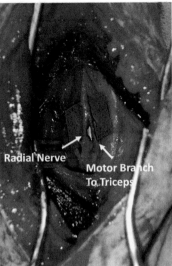

Fig. 5. The posterior approach to TMR in the transhumeral amputee. TMR of the radial nerve to a motor branch of the triceps is performed from this approach.

Partial Hand Amputee

Recently, TMR has been described for treatment of neuroma pain after an amputated digit.[36] Volarly, neuromas of the transected digital nerves can be identified and coapted to motor branches to the palmar and/or dorsal interosseus muscles (**Fig. 8**). It is important to confirm with nerve stimulation that the motor branch to the interosseus muscle goes to an expendable muscle and not one to the residual digits. On the dorsal aspect, patients can present with neuromas of the superficial branch of the radial nerve (dorsoradial aspect of hand) or to the dorsal branch of the ulnar nerve (dorsoulnar aspect of hand), which may be amenable to TMR to the dorsal interossei motor branches. Alternatively, more proximal transection of the superficial branch of the radial nerve with coaptation to a posterior interosseus motor nerve branch has been described.[36]

Above-Knee Amputee

TMR for the above-knee amputee can target the tibial nerve, common peroneal nerve, and posterior cutaneous nerve of the thigh through a single posterior thigh incision. An alternate anteriomedial incision can be made if needed to treat the saphenous nerve or lateral femoral cutaneous nerve of the thigh (**Table 4**).

Regardless of whether TMR is performed in delayed or immediate fashion, the authors find it is best to perform TMR for the above-knee amputee in a prone position through a single posterior thigh incision, separate from the incision required for osteotomy (**Fig. 9**). This incision starts distally at about 50% of original thigh length (using the contralateral intact leg to measure thigh length from ischium to popliteal fossa).[37] The incision extends from 50% thigh length to about 6 to 8 cm proximal. This incision is roughly at the junction

Table 3
Example pattern of targeted muscle reinnervation nerve transfers in a transradial amputee

Donor Nerve	Recipient Nerve	Muscle Innervated	Special Considerations
Median	Anterior interosseus	flexor pollicis longus, FDP to index and long fingers	
Ulnar	Ulnar motor branch	FCU	
Superficial branch of radial nerve	Radial motor branch	Brachioradialis	
LABC	Median motor branch	FCR	
MABC	Ulnar motor branch	FCU	

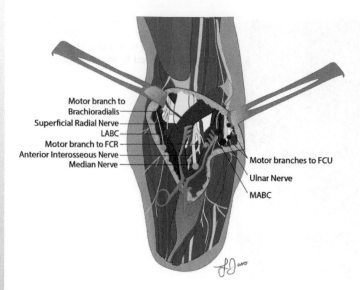

Fig. 6. Approach to TMR for transradial amputees. Median nerve to AIN (*blue dots*), ulnar nerve to motor branch to FCU (*black dots*), MABC to motor branch to FCU (*purple dots*), LABC to motor branch to FCR (*green dots*), superficial radial nerve to motor branch to brachioradialis (*pink dots*). FCU, flexor carpi ulnaris; FCR, flexor carpi radialis.

between the proximal and middle thirds of the thigh. It is often helpful to compare the residual limb length to the contralateral thigh for comparison. The sciatic nerve is identified in the space between the rectus femoris and semitendinosus. Neurolysis is performed to separate it into tibial and common peroneal components. The tibial nerve is coapted to a motor branch to the semitendinosus while the common peroneal nerve is coapted to a branch to the biceps femoris. The posterior cutaneous nerve of the thigh can be coapted to a motor branch to either of these,

depending on what is available in closest proximity with least tension.

The saphenous nerve can be targeted via an incision approximately 10 cm proximal to the medial femoral condyle (using the contralateral leg as a reference). It can be found exiting between the sartorius and gracilis tendons at this level and traced proximally into the adductor canal until a motor branch to the vastus medialis is identified as a recipient. The lateral femoral cutaneous nerve of the thigh can be found through the same incision used for an anterolateral thigh flap approach

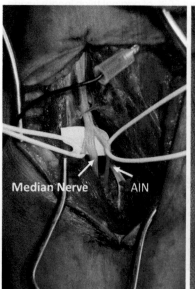
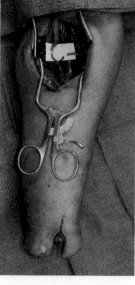

Fig. 7. TMR through single incision in transradial amputee. TMR for the hand. TMR of digital nerves to hypothenar motor branches.

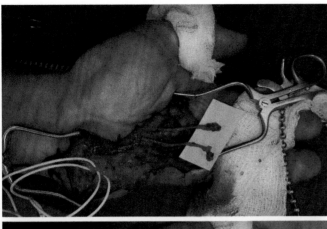
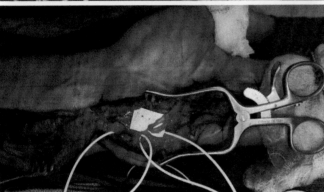

Fig. 8. Example TMR for the hand. TMR of digital nerves to hypothenar motor branches.

and can be targeted to a motor branch to the vastus lateralis.

Below-Knee Amputee

Many variations exist for TMR in the below-knee amputee, depending on whether it is performed in immediate or delayed fashion and whether it is performed through a 1- or 2-incision approach (**Tables 5 and 6**).[38] Nerves to consider in the below-knee amputee include the common peroneal (with deep and superficial divisions), the tibial, the saphenous, and the medial and lateral sural nerves.

It is possible to perform TMR acutely at the time of amputation through the open amputation site with a proximal lateral extension to access the peroneal nerve branches. A nerve stimulator is particularly useful in these cases, as the anatomy is distorted. Each nerve ending is tagged with a hemostat and dissected proximally for length. Adjacent motor targets are identified with a nerve stimulator. Coaptations are then performed between the distal nerve ends and the transected motor branches.

Alternatively, below-knee TMR can be performed in delayed fashion. A 2-incision approach

Table 4
Example pattern of targeted muscle reinnervation nerve transfers in an above-knee amputee

Donor Nerve	Recipient Nerve	Muscle Innervated	Special Considerations
Common peroneal	Sciatic motor branch	Biceps femoris long head	Whether performed acutely at the time of amputation or in delayed fashion, the authors recommend approaching through a separate single incision in the posterior thigh
Tibial	Sciatic motor branch	Semitendinosis	
Posterior cutaneous	Sciatic motor branch	Semitendinosis or biceps femoris	
Lateral femoral cutaneous	Femoral motor branch	Vastus lateralis	
Saphenous	Femoral motor branch	Vastus medialis	

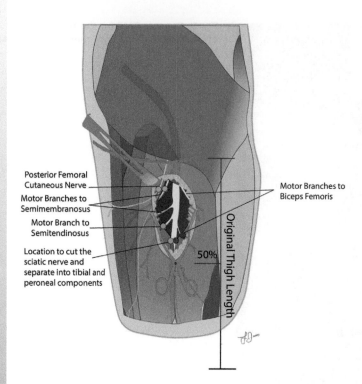

Fig. 9. Approach to TMR for Above Knee Amputees. Tibial nerve to motor branch to semitendinosus (*green dots*), peroneal nerve to motor branch to biceps femoris (*pink dots*), posterior femoral cutaneous nerve to motor branch to semimembranosus (*blue dots*), (saphenous nerve to vastus medialis can be performed through the amputation incision when the patient in supine).

Posterior Femoral Cutaneous Nerve

Motor Branches to Semimembranosus

Motor Branch to Semitendinosus

Location to cut the sciatic nerve and separate into tibial and peroneal components

Motor Branches to Biceps Femoris

Original Thigh Length

50%

uses an anterolateral incision for identification of deep and superficial peroneal nerve branches and a posterior calf incision for the tibial and sural nerve branches, performed in the lateral decubitus position or using a supine/prone position change. The advantage of this 2-incision approach is that it retains some native anterior compartment innervation by performing TMR to the most distal available peroneal nerve targets, thereby retaining some residual limb soft tissue bulk. The other option is to do the entire procedure through a single posterior calf ("stocking seam") incision in the prone position, targeting the common peroneal, tibial, and sural nerves all to gastrocnemius and soleus motor branches (**Fig. 10**). When performing TMR through a single incision, effort should still be made to perform an intrafascicular dissection of the common peroneal nerve to isolate and preserve some proximal motor fascicles to the anterior and lateral compartments for muscle bulk. The single-incision technique results in faster operating time, negates the need for a patient flip, but may result in a greater amount of anterior and lateral compartment muscle denervation if motor branches are not preserved.

NONAMPUTEES

TMR is a reliable technique to treat chronic neuroma pain when neuroma excision and nerve reconstruction either are not possible or have failed. Nonamputee patients present more often

---

Table 5
Example pattern of targeted muscle reinnervation nerve transfers in a below-knee amputee through a single incision approach

Donor Nerve	Recipient Nerve	Muscle Innervated	Special Considerations
Common peroneal	Tibial motor branch	Lateral gastrocnemius	This approach eliminates the need for a patient flip midoperation, but may result in a greater amount of denervation atrophy to the anterior and lateral compartment musculature
Tibial	Tibial motor branch	Soleus	
Medial sural	Tibial motor branch	Medial gastrocnemius	
Lateral sural	Tibial motor branch	Lateral gastrocnemius	

Table 6
Example pattern of targeted muscle reinnervation nerve transfers in a below-knee amputee through a dual incision approach with a patient flip

Donor Nerve	Recipient Nerve	Muscle Innervated	Special Considerations
Deep peroneal	Peroneal motor branch	Tibialis anterior or extensor digitorum longus	This approach requires a patient flip midoperation, but may be beneficial in preserving some native innervation to the anterior and lateral compartment musculature
Superficial peroneal	Peroneal motor branch	Peroneus longus	
Tibial	Tibial motor branch	Soleus	
Medial sural	Tibial motor branch	Medial gastrocnemius	
Lateral sural	Tibial motor branch	Lateral gastrocnemius	

with neuromas-in-continuity because of either compression, trauma, or prior surgery rather than end neuromas. It is common to find incision scars overlying the area where patients complain of the greatest tenderness, indicating a likely neuroma.

Common extremity presentations include superficial radial neuroma after chronic compression, trauma, or wrist surgery; superficial peroneal, saphenous, and or sural neuromas after foot and ankle surgery (**Fig. 11**); and saphenous neuroma in the thigh after knee arthroscopy or total knee arthroplasty. Recommended incisions and targets have been previously detailed and are outlined in **Table 7**.[6,7,38]

TMR is often thought of as extremity surgery; however, any patient who presents with chronic nerve-type pain in a specific distribution should be considered for TMR. For example, TMR has been described for the treatment of

postmastectomy pain with transfer of the cut breast intercostal nerves to serratus anterior, intercostal, or pectoral muscles.[39] At the authors' institution, they have effectively treated occipital neuromas with refractory migraine pain after decompression and/or neuroma excision and grafting with TMR to the splenius capitus (**Fig. 12**). In addition, patients presenting with groin pain after abdominal or hernia surgery have been successfully treated with TMR of the ilioinguinal and/or genitofemoral nerves to a motor nerve of the internal oblique.

The approach to these patients is to (1) mark the area of greatest Tinel preoperatively; (2) design a 3- to 4-cm incision overlying this area; (3) dissect to the anatomic tissue plane where the neuroma is expected; (4) continue dissection in this plane until the abnormal neuroma tissue is identified (often palpation of the area for firm/abnormal

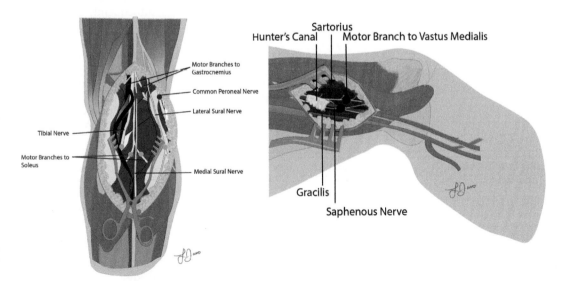

Fig. 10. Approach to TMR for Below Knee Amputees. Tibial nerve to motor branch to medial soleus (*green dots*), common peroneal nerve to motor branch to lateral gastrocnemius (*purple dots*), lateral sural nerve to motor branch to lateral soleus (blue dots, medial sural neve to medial branch to gastrocnemius (*pink dots*), saphenous nerve to motor branch to vastus medialis (*black dots*).

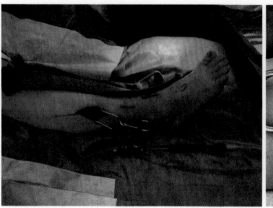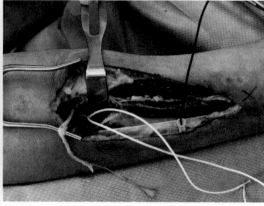

Fig. 11. Example TMR for neuroma in continuity in non-amputee, deep peroneal sensory branch to EDC motor branch. EDC, extensor digitorum communis.

Table 7			
Techniques summary for common neuroma patterns in non- amputees			
	Common Sources of Injury	**Recommended Nerve Targets**	**Incision Placement**
Superficial radial neuroma	Compression (Wartenberg syndrome) Trauma Wrist surgery	Brachioradialis Extensor carpi radialis brevis	4-5 cm starting 9 cm proximal to radial styloid and extending proximally
Medial antebrachial cutaneous neuroma	Ulnar nerve decompression Elbow surgery Brachioplasty	Flexor carpi ulnaris	10-cm V-shaped incision that follows along the course of the pronator teres, apexes over the medial epicondyle, and subsequently courses toward the biceps
Lateral antebrachial cutaneous neuroma	Elbow surgery	Flexor carpi radialis	8 cm along the volar midline just distal to the antecubital fossa
Saphenous neuroma	Arthroscopic knee surgery Ankle surgery	Vastus medialis gracilis	6-8 cm starting 10 cm proximal to the medial femoral condyle extending along the posterior axis of the femur
Superficial peroneal neuroma	Compression neuroma Ankle surgery	Peroneus longus	6-8 cm along a line drawn from lateral femoral condyle to lateral malleolus between 20% and −40% of leg length
Deep peroneal neuroma	Ankle surgery	Extensor digitorum longus	6-8 cm parallel and 1 cm lateral to tibia between 50% and −70% of leg length
Sural neuroma	Ankle surgery	Gastrocnemius	6-8 cm along posterior midline between 10% and −20% of leg length

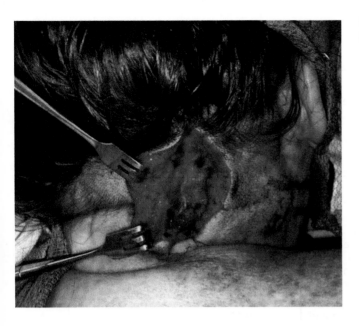

Fig. 12. Example TMR for neuroma of occipital nerve.

tissue is helpful to guide discovery); (5) use a nerve stimulator to locate adjacent motor nerves for coaptation; and finally, (6) perform TMR nerve coaptation and close.

DISCUSSION

Residual limb pain and phantom limb pain are well-known sequelae of major extremity amputation. TMR is a successful technique for the treatment of chronic phantom limb pain,[5] and TMR at the time of amputation significantly reduces the incidence and severity of phantom limb pain and residual limb pain compared with cross-sectional controls.[9] It has similarly been shown to treat neuroma pain, specifically.[4]

Although TMR can be performed for any nerve, there are several overarching principles that apply to most cases. For instance, if one is having difficulty identifying a recipient motor nerve, it is often possible to dissect the main donor nerve trunk proximally to identify a motor branch coming off this main nerve trunk. In this way, the donor nerve gets transferred to its own motor branch. Second, it is important to be able to identify potential recipient motor nerve branches with nerve stimulation. As such, the authors typically do not use regional anesthesia in these cases and generally opt for general anesthesia. They also like to limit tourniquet time to less than 40 minutes to prevent dampening of nerve conduction signals, which can in turn make it more difficult to identify motor branches. Last, most cases of TMR involve the transfer of a larger donor nerve to a much smaller motor branch. The authors have not found nerve size mismatch to be an issue with this technique, unlike when performing nerve transfers for functional muscle recovery where precise coaptation is more crucial. To deal with the nerve size mismatch, the authors essentially intussuscept the smaller recipient nerve into the larger donor nerve with 1 to 2 polypropylene sutures. They then will suture the donor epineurium to adjacent epimysium to take tension off the coaptation and secure it in place.

Most importantly, it is important for the surgeon to remain flexible during TMR, using adjacent recipient nerve motor branches that are available rather than relying on precise, predetermined transfer patterns. The available pattern of recipient motor nerves can vary significantly from patient to patient and is dependent on amputation level, soft tissue deficits, and other nerve injury patterns.

SUMMARY

TMR is a surgical technique that has demonstrated success for the treatment of residual limb pain and phantom limb pain in amputees, and it can similarly treat neuroma pain in the nonamputee. Although the exact pattern of nerve transfers is variable, the key principle that will determine success with TMR is finding an appropriate recipient motor nerve branch that the proximal portion of the neuromatous nerve can be coapted to in a tension-free manner. By relying on the principle of giving the nerve "somewhere to go and something to do," TMR provides a way of reconstructing the otherwise un-reconstructable nerve.

CLINICS CARE POINTS

- When evaluating a patient for targeted muscle reinnervation, be sure to elicit muscle contraction of potential recipient motor nerve muscle groups to determine what targets are available.

- Avoid the use of local or regional anesthetic and limit tourniquet time to make it easier to identify potential motor nerve recipients with a nerve stimulator.

- Nerve coaptation often involves a size discrepancy between donor and recipient nerves. The authors have not found this to be a problem and deal with this by intussuscepting the smaller recipient nerve into the larger donor nerve.

- The pattern of nerve transfers is variable and can differ from patient to patient, depending on surgeon preference, patient-specific anatomy, amputation level, and other deficits. Here, the authors provide transfer patterns that they have found work well, but targeted muscle reinnervation often requires some degree of flexibility.

DISCLOSURE

Drs J.H. Ko and G.A. Dumanian are on the Scientific Advisory Board of Checkpoint Surgical, Inc. Dr G.A. Dumanian is founder of the Advanced Suture Inc and the Mesh Suture Inc. Dr J.H. Ko is a consultant for Integra LifeSciences Corporation.

REFERENCES

1. Alviar MJ, Hale T, Dungca M. Pharmacologic interventions for treating phantom limb pain. Cochrane Database Syst Rev 2011;(12):Cd006380.
2. Huse E, Larbig W, Flor H, et al. The effect of opioids on phantom limb pain and cortical reorganization. Pain 2001;90(1–2):47–55.
3. Gilron I, Bailey JM, Tu D, et al. Morphine, gabapentin, or their combination for neuropathic pain. N Engl J Med 2005;352(13):1324–34.
4. Souza JM, Cheesborough JE, Ko JH, et al. Targeted muscle reinnervation: a novel approach to postamputation neuroma pain. Clin Orthopa Relat Res 2014;472(10):2984–90.
5. Dumanian GA, Potter BK, Mioton LM, et al. Targeted muscle reinnervation treats neuroma and phantom pain in major limb amputees: a randomized clinical trial. Ann Surg 2019;270(2):238–46.
6. Janes LE, Fracol ME, Ko JH, et al. Management of unreconstructable saphenous nerve injury with targeted muscle reinnervation. Plast Reconstr Surg Glob Open 2020;8(1):e2383.
7. Fracol ME, Dumanian GA, Janes LE, et al. Management of sural nerve neuromas with targeted muscle reinnervation. Plast Reconstr Surg Glob Open 2020; 8(1):e2545.
8. Cheesborough JE, Souza JM, Dumanian GA, et al. Targeted muscle reinnervation in the initial management of traumatic upper extremity amputation injury. Hand (N Y) 2014;9(2):253–7.
9. Valerio IL, Dumanian GA, Jordan SW, et al. Preemptive treatment of phantom and residual limb pain with targeted muscle reinnervation at the time of major limb amputation. J Am Coll Surg 2019;228(3): 217–26.
10. Smith DG, Ehde DM, Legro MW, et al. Phantom limb, residual limb, and back pain after lower extremity amputations. Clin Orthop Relat Res 1999;(361): 29–38.
11. Ephraim PL, Wegener ST, MacKenzie EJ, et al. Phantom pain, residual limb pain, and back pain in amputees: results of a national survey. Arch Phys Med Rehabil 2005;86(10):1910–9.
12. Pierce RO Jr, Kernek CB, Ambrose TA 2nd. The plight of the traumatic amputee. Orthopedics 1993; 16(7):793–7.
13. Hanley MA, Ehde DM, Jensen M, et al. Chronic pain associated with upper-limb loss. Am J Phys Med Rehabil 2009;88(9):742–51 [quiz: 752, 779].
14. Fisher K, Hanspal RS, Marks L. Return to work after lower limb amputation. Int J Rehabil Res 2003;26(1): 51–6.
15. Schoppen T, Boonstra A, Groothoff JW, et al. Employment status, job characteristics, and work-related health experience of people with a lower limb amputation in The Netherlands. Arch Phys Med Rehabil 2001;82(2):239–45.
16. Raichle KA, Hanley MA, Molton I, et al. Prosthesis use in persons with lower- and upper-limb amputation. J Rehabil Res Dev 2008;45(7): 961–72.
17. Dolezal JM, Vernick SH, Khan N, et al. Factors associated with use and nonuse of an AK prosthesis in a rural, southern, geriatric population. Int J Rehabil Health 1998;4(4):245–51.
18. Hagberg K, Brånemark R. Consequences of nonvascular trans-femoral amputation: a survey of quality of life, prosthetic use and problems. Prosthetics Orthotics Int 2001;25(3):186–94.
19. Tintle SM, Baechler MF, Nanos GP, et al. Reoperations following combat-related upper-extremity amputations. J Bone Joint Surg Am 2012;94(16):e1191–6.
20. Sheehan TP, Gondo GC. Impact of limb loss in the United States. Phys Med Rehabil Clin N Am 2014; 25(1):9–28.

21. Geraghty TJ, Jones LE. Painful neuromata following upper limb amputation. Prosthetics orthotics Int 1996;20(3):176–81.

22. Rajput K, Reddy S, Shankar H. Painful neuromas. Clin J Pain 2012;28(7):639–45.

23. Macrae WA. Chronic pain after surgery. Br J Anaesth 2001;87(1):88–98.

24. Sarris I, Gobel F, Gainer M, et al. Medial brachial and antebrachial cutaneous nerve injuries: effect on outcome in revision cubital tunnel surgery. J Reconstr microsurgery 2002;18(8):665–70.

25. Louis DS, Greene TL, Noellert RC. Complications of carpal tunnel surgery. J Neurosurg 1985;62(3):352–6.

26. Dellon AL, Mackinnon SE. Susceptibility of the superficial sensory branch of the radial nerve to form painful neuromas. J Hand Surg Br 1984;9(1):42–5.

27. Kuiken TA, Dumanian GA, Lipschutz RD, et al. The use of targeted muscle reinnervation for improved myoelectric prosthesis control in a bilateral shoulder disarticulation amputee. Prosthetics orthotics Int 2004;28(3):245–53.

28. Kuiken TA, Miller LA, Lipschutz RD, et al. Targeted reinnervation for enhanced prosthetic arm function in a woman with a proximal amputation: a case study. Lancet 2007;369(9559):371–80.

29. Farina D, Castronovo AM, Vujaklija I, et al. Common synaptic input to motor neurons and neural drive to targeted reinnervated muscles. J Neurosci 2017;37(46):11285–92.

30. Kim PS, Ko JH, O'Shaughnessy KK, et al. The effects of targeted muscle reinnervation on neuromas in a rabbit rectus abdominis flap model. J Hand Surg 2012;37(8):1609–16.

31. Guse DM, Moran SL. Outcomes of the surgical treatment of peripheral neuromas of the hand and forearm: a 25-year comparative outcome study. Ann Plast Surg 2013;71(6):654–8.

32. Souza JM, Purnell CA, Cheesborough JE, et al. Treatment of foot and ankle neuroma pain with processed nerve allografts. Foot Ankle Int 2016;37(10):1098–105.

33. Gart MS, Souza JM, Dumanian GA. Targeted muscle reinnervation in the upper extremity amputee: a technical roadmap. J Hand Surg 2015;40(9):1877–88.

34. Daly MC, He JJ, Ponton RP, et al. A single incision anterior approach for transhumeral amputation targeted muscle reinnervation. Plast Reconstr Surg Glob Open 2020;8(4):e2750.

35. Morgan EN, Kyle Potter B, Souza JM, et al. Targeted muscle reinnervation for transradial amputation: description of operative technique. Tech Hand Upper Extremity Surg 2016;20(4):166–71.

36. Daugherty THF, Bueno RA Jr, Neumeister MW. Novel use of targeted muscle reinnervation in the hand for treatment of recurrent symptomatic neuromas following digit amputations. Plast Reconstr Surg Glob open 2019;7(8):e2376.

37. Agnew SP, Schultz AE, Dumanian GA, et al. Targeted reinnervation in the transfemoral amputee: a preliminary study of surgical technique. Plast Reconstr Surg 2012;129(1):187–94.

38. Fracol ME, Janes LE, Ko JH, et al. Targeted muscle reinnervation in the lower leg: an anatomical study. Plast Reconstr Surg 2018;142(4):541e–50e.

39. O'Brien AL, Kraft CT, Valerio IL, et al. Targeted muscle reinnervation following breast surgery: a novel technique. Plast Reconstr Surg Glob Open 2020;8(4):e2782.

Regenerative Peripheral Nerve Interfaces for the Treatment and Prevention of Neuromas and Neuroma Pain

Nishant Ganesh Kumar, MD, Theodore A. Kung, MD*

KEYWORDS

- Amputation • Neuroma • Regenerative peripheral nerve interface • RPNI • Prosthetic control
- Phantom limb pain • Neuroma pain • Residual limb pain

KEY POINTS

- A neuroma occurs when a regenerating peripheral nerve has no distal target. Aimless axonal regeneration leads to ectopic neural activity that results in debilitating pain and functional limitations.
- Pain from neuromas can lead to centralization of peripheral neuropathic pain and exacerbation of symptoms. In addition, neuroma pain can contribute to depression, anxiety, opioid dependence, poor prosthetic compliance, and delayed prosthetic rehabilitation among affected individuals.
- Many noninvasive and surgical treatment strategies exist to treat neuromas. Most commonly, surgical intervention for neuroma pain involves excision of the symptomatic neuroma and implantation of the nerve in adjacent muscle or bone. However, outcomes from this approach are inconsistent and do not attempt to mitigate the propensity for neuroma recurrence.
- The regenerative peripheral nerve interface (RPNI) is a simple, robust, safe, and clinically proven technique to prevent the formation of neuromas and treat existing symptomatic neuromas. In addition, RPNIs can be used for high-fidelity prosthetic control of the upper and lower extremity.

INTRODUCTION

Neuromas are a manifestation of aimless and disorganized neural regeneration that occurs after transection of a peripheral nerve without repair and can be symptomatic or asymptomatic.[1,2] Symptomatic neuromas have been reported after a variety of operations, such as limb amputation, mastectomy, abdominal wall surgery, head and neck surgery, foot and ankle surgery, and orthognathic surgery.[3–8] Classically, symptomatic neuromas are characterized by pain that can be burning, sharp, or associated with tingling sensations.[2] Symptomatic neuroma pain is frequently experienced after major limb amputation and is associated with considerable morbidity.

Pain after major limb amputation, or postamputation pain, affects hundreds of thousands of individuals, with reported rates as high as 75% to 80% among patients with amputation.[8–12] Postamputation pain is multifactorial and consists of phantom limb pain and residual limb pain.[8] Phantom limb pain refers to pain in the distribution of the amputated part, whereas residual limb pain refers to pain localized within the residual limb and includes neuroma pain.[8] Although a variety of peripheral, spinal, and supraspinal alterations have been studied and implicated in the mechanisms behind postamputation pain, it is still not completely understood.[13–17] Neuropathic pain after amputation from traumatic symptomatic neuromas can have significant emotional and psychological effects

Section of Plastic Surgery, Department of Surgery, University of Michigan, 1500 East Medical Center Drive, 2130 Taubman Center, Ann Arbor, MI 48109-5231, USA
* Corresponding author.
E-mail address: thekung@med.umich.edu

Hand Clin 37 (2021) 361–371
https://doi.org/10.1016/j.hcl.2021.05.003
0749-0712/21/© 2021 Elsevier Inc. All rights reserved.

contributing to depression and anxiety.[18,19] Furthermore, many individuals resort to chronic opioid use to cope with postamputation neuropathic pain.[20] Therefore, there remains a need to treat preexisting postamputation pain and prevent the development of recurrent postamputation pain.

Because neuromas contribute to the manifestation of postamputation pain, many nonoperative and operative strategies have been described to manage symptomatic neuromas. However, there is still no gold standard procedure to effectively treat symptomatic neuromas or to prevent the formation of symptomatic neuromas. This article provides an overview of management strategies for patients with symptomatic neuromas and focuses on the regenerative peripheral nerve interface (RPNI) as a surgical strategy to treat and prevent postamputation pain.

PRESENTATION AND DIAGNOSIS

Following injury to a peripheral nerve, the distal axonal segment undergoes wallerian degeneration and the proximal axonal segment undergoes sprouting and regeneration.[21,22] The end goal of the regenerating peripheral nerve is to attempt to reinnervate a distal target. However, when this process is interrupted or unsuccessful, such as in the case of amputation injury without repair, the terminal peripheral nerve inevitably forms a disorganized mass of regenerating axons and scar tissue that constitutes an end neuroma (**Fig. 1**).[23,24] On histology, neuromas show perineural cells and fascicles encased in dense fibrous tissue resulting from proliferation of local fibroblasts, macrophages, myofibroblasts, and perineural cells.[23,25] Within these disorganized neural bundles, there is an upregulation of sodium channels that contributes to ectopic activity and exacerbates the characteristic neuropathic pain associated with neuromas.[26–28] Clinically, this sequence of events contributes to some of the classic symptoms patients present with: sharp shooting sensations, burning pain, low-temperature intolerance, paresthesias, numbness, and hypersensitivity.[29,30] In addition, patients with amputations experiencing neuroma pain may also have considerable difficulty with prosthetic rehabilitation and prolonged prosthetic use.[31] Patients who pursue surgical treatment of neuromas often present with these distinctive symptoms and complaints.

During the evaluation of symptomatic neuromas, attention to the timing, duration, and onset of symptoms should be recorded because most neuromas develop 6 to 10 weeks after surgery.[1] The diagnosis of a symptomatic neuroma is made clinically with solicitation of point tenderness with percussion at a specific site (Tinel sign). Diagnostic confirmation can be performed by injection of a local anesthetic at the site of maximal point tenderness resulting in alleviation of symptoms. Such a response suggests that surgical intervention is likely to be favorable.[1,32] If imaging is desired for better neuroma localization, ultrasonography and MRI studies are the preferred modalities, although use of computed tomography scans has also been reported.[33–37]

In treating patients with neuroma pain, it is important for clinicians to be cognizant of central neurologic processes that may be potentiating a patient's pain experience. After peripheral nerve injury, patients often report peripheral neuropathic pain, which has been associated with centrally mediated phenomena such as depression, posttraumatic stress disorder, catastrophizing, and phantom limb pain.[38,39] In addition, peripheral neuropathic pain can cause central neuropathic pain or central sensitization. Central sensitization represents changes in the properties of neurons in the central nervous system that result in central neuronal hyperexcitability and reduced inhibition.[40] Because the centralization is caused by changes in the properties of neurons, pain is no longer coupled to the intensity, presence, or duration of acute peripheral nociceptive inputs. Instead, centralization represents pain caused by enhanced central neuronal activity and hypersensitivity despite subthreshold synaptic inputs.[40] Clinically, the central nervous system responds as if there is a state of persistent pain and hypersensitivity to pain despite limited peripheral input.[41–43] Centralization of pain can occur when acute pain persists and becomes chronic, and can occur when a person develops a peripheral pain state.[41] For instance, chronic back pain is considered an example of peripheral pain that can become centralized.[41] It is important to recognize central sensitization resulting from peripheral nerve injury because interventions designed to ameliorate peripheral pain may not be as effective if centralization has occurred.[44] Furthermore, in spite of evidence-based interventions to treat neuroma pain, central sensitization likely plays a role in sustaining postoperative residual limb pain in some patients.[45] It is for these reasons that a comprehensive approach that targets peripheral and central processes to treating postamputation pain is necessary. Therefore, in addition to treatment of the peripheral source of pain, treatment of central pain through the use of neuromodulators, antiepileptics, and antidepressants should be considered.[41]

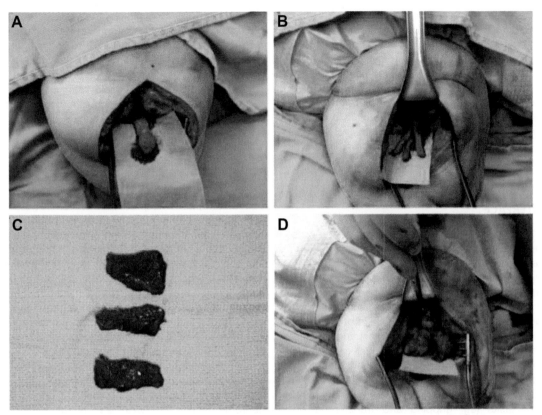

Fig. 1. Excision of sciatic nerve neuroma and creation of fascicular RPNIs. (*A*) Identification of sciatic nerve end neuroma. (*B*) After excision of neuroma and transecting nerve at the level of healthy-appearing fascicles, meticulous dissection is performed to divide the nerve into 3 distinct fascicles. (*C*) Autologous free skeletal muscle grafts are harvested from the biceps femoris muscle. (*D*) RPNIs are performed by securing each fascicle of the sciatic nerve within a separate skeletal muscle graft. (*From* Woo SL, Kung TA, Brown DL, Leonard JA, Kelly BM, Cederna PS. Regenerative Peripheral Nerve Interfaces for the Treatment of Postamputation Neuroma Pain: A Pilot Study. Plast Reconstr Surg Glob Open. 2016;4(12):e1038.)

TREATMENT

Many treatment strategies have been proposed to treat neuroma pain. These strategies range from less invasive techniques such as desensitization, transcutaneous electrical stimulation, local injections of anesthetics, and pharmacotherapy, to more invasive ones that involve surgical intervention such as neuroma excision, capping, and transposition into bone, muscle, or vein.[46–55] In spite of these proposed solutions, no method is widely adopted because of variability in outcomes and high rates of neuroma recurrence.[56] A recent meta-analysis has shown that surgical treatment of neuroma pain may be effective in 77% of patients, with no significant difference seen among surgical techniques.[57] Therefore no single surgical technique is considered the gold standard in the surgical treatment of neuroma pain. Nevertheless, surgical treatment of neuromas is frequently pursued because it has been shown to improve patient-reported pain, phantom limb pain, depression, and quality of life.[58,59]

One of the most popular surgical techniques for neuroma management is the technique published by Dellon and Mackinnon[47] in the 1980s. This technique involved neuroma excision and placement of the end of the residual nerve in a location away from denervated skin, away from tension, and buried into the well-vascularized environment of local innervated muscle. Although this technique provides soft tissue cushioning around the cut nerve end, it does not provide any targets for reinnervation and therefore there is inevitable recurrence of the neuroma, although this may be less symptomatic simply because it has reformed in a less problematic location. Eberlin and Ducic[56] noted that, when considering surgical interventions for neuroma management, there are procedures that are "passive/ablative" and those that are "active/reconstructive." Neuroma excision and implantation into already-innervated tissue is considered a passive technique because it does not address the prevention of neuroma formation. In contrast, active methods such as primary nerve repair, hollow tube reconstruction, allograft or autograft reconstruction, targeted muscle reinnervation (TMR), and RPNIs are considered to be more physiologic in preventing neuroma pain by allowing regenerating axons the ability to reinnervate, thereby reducing the number of aimless axons that subsequently contribute to neuroma formation.[56,60]

THE REGENERATIVE PERIPHERAL NERVE INTERFACE

The RPNI was initially described as a neuroprosthetic control strategy and comprises a residual peripheral nerve or an individual nerve fascicle implanted into an autologous free skeletal muscle graft. Fascicular RPNIs of major peripheral nerves in the upper extremity (eg, median, ulnar, and radial) have been used as amplifiers of peripheral nerve signals to control an artificial hand after upper extremity amputation.[61–63] Specifically, RPNIs have been implanted in humans to enable continuous finger movement of a prosthetic hand in real time for 300 days to complete a variety of human tasks (eg, gripping and transferring objects).[64] Before its use in humans, extensive laboratory studies in animal models showed the presence of axonal sprouting, elongation, and synaptogenesis within the RPNI.[65] In addition to showing the formation of new neuromuscular junctions, these studies also confirmed the absence of formation of new neuromas and the stability of RPNIs over time. In nonhuman primate studies, RPNIs have remained stable and viable for up to 20 months postimplantation.[66]

To perform RPNI surgery, autologous free skeletal muscle grafts are used (**Fig. 2**). Initially, these free skeletal muscle grafts are both devascularized and denervated. Once a skeletal muscle graft is secured around the terminal end of a peripheral nerve, each skeletal muscle graft undergoes the physiologic processes of regeneration, revascularization, and reinnervation.[67–69] As with any tissue graft, survival of the muscle graft is contingent on a well-described process of imbibition, inosculation, and revascularization. Therefore, adequate vascular perfusion to the wound bed is critical to prevent central necrosis of the muscle graft and potential failure of the RPNI. As it undergoes revascularization, the denervated muscle provides an immediate local reinnervation target for the distal end of the transected peripheral nerve. This reinnervation of the skeletal muscle graft by the implanted peripheral nerve forms

new neuromuscular junctions and prevents the disorganized, purposeless axonal sprouting associated with neuromas. Thus, the RPNI can mitigate neuroma pain by lessening the propensity for neuroma formation. This phenomenon of synaptogenesis within the skeletal muscle graft leading to successful reinnervation distinguishes the RPNI neuroma strategy from the technique of burying a residual nerve into local innervated muscle.

Reinnervation of denervated muscle to reduce neuroma formation is also central to the efficacy of TMR to treat neuroma pain.[70] TMR was also conceived as a way to foster improved intuitive control of upper-limb prosthetic limbs. However, TMR uses the technique of multiple nerve transfers to reroute donor axons to reinnervate purposefully denervated portions of local muscle.[71–75] Briefly, the TMR technique involves division of a motor nerve to an expendable segment of skeletal muscle to create a denervated target. The end of a transected peripheral nerve is then transferred and coapted to the selected recipient motor nerve in order to reinnervate this denervated skeletal muscle.[56,76] Experimentally, this has been shown to be effective in minimizing neuroma formation.[77,78] Similar to RPNI surgery, TMR has shown success in clinical settings to prevent and treat neuroma pain as well as phantom limb pain.[59,76,79] Because both these techniques minimize the incidence of symptomatic neuroma formation, they can prevent the maladaptive process of central sensitization. This ability in turn may explain the efficacy of such physiologic techniques in decreasing peripheral neuroma pain in addition to minimizing centrally mediated phantom limb pain.[80]

Mechanistically, TMR and RPNI involve similar approaches in that a peripheral nerve is provided with denervated muscle tissue to encourage the formation of new neuromuscular junctions to minimize neuroma formation. However, there are some key differences between these techniques. TMR requires nerve transfer techniques that frequently involve the coaptation of 2 nerves with a considerable size mismatch. For instance, common nerve transfers in TMR after upper extremity amputation include transfer of the large residual median nerve to the significantly smaller motor nerve of the short head of the biceps brachii and transfer of the large distal radial nerve to the significantly smaller motor nerve of the lateral head of the triceps.[81] Such a size discrepancy during coaptation is a known risk factor for neuroma in continuity at the site of the repair.[82] In addition, the proximal aspect of the sacrificed motor nerve is shortened and moved away from the coaptation site to prevent it from contributing to reinnervation, which has been

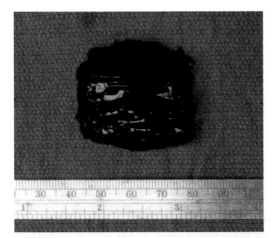

Fig. 2. Free skeletal muscle graft harvested from donor skeletal muscle. Skeletal muscle grafts typically measure 30 to 40 mm long, 15 to 20 mm wide, and 5 to 6 mm thick. (*From* Santosa KB, Oliver JD, Cederna PS, Kung TA. Regenerative Peripheral Nerve Interfaces for Prevention and Management of Neuromas. Clin Plast Surg. 2020;47(2):311-321.)

observed.[81] Although it is possible that this sacrificed motor nerve does not form a symptomatic neuroma, it is unclear whether this motor nerve neuroma could still contribute to centrally mediated pain processes, as previously discussed. In contrast, RPNI surgery does not involve nerve transfer techniques nor does it involve the formation of new neuromas originating from sacrificed motor nerves. Each RPNI takes about 7 to 10 minutes to successfully complete and does not require the tedious identification and dissection of donor motor nerve branches.[83] However, the success of RPNIs is contingent on correct technique, which involves obtaining muscle grafts of an appropriate thickness and size to match the size of the peripheral nerve or nerve fascicle, and creating RPNIs in a wound bed that is well vascularized.

OPERATIVE PEARLS TO PERFORM REGENERATIVE PERIPHERAL NERVE INTERFACE SURGERY

Any patient being considered for surgical treatment of a neuroma must have a thorough preoperative work-up for all contributing sources of postamputation pain (eg, heterotopic ossification, infection, bone spurs). For instance, imaging may reveal additional causes of residual limb pain, such as infection, fracture, malunion, and heterotopic ossification.[84] Preoperative identification of these diagnoses is imperative because they may contribute to persistent postoperative pain. For

instance, heterotopic ossification is seen in up to 60% of patients who undergo amputation[85] and can contribute to inadequate pain relief for patients that undergo neuroma management alone.[86,87] Similarly, for patients with multiple neuromas seen on imaging, treatment of the most symptomatic neuroma may unmask other less symptomatic neuromas. To optimize outcomes, surgical intervention is considered for all symptomatic neuromas to reduce the chances of persistent pain resulting from unmasked symptomatic neuromas.

RPNI surgery is easy to perform and reproducible. When used to treat neuroma pain, the patient is asked preoperatively to point at the site of maximal tenderness, and this is marked to serve as a guide for where the symptomatic neuroma may be located. Intraoperatively, careful and meticulous dissection is required to adequately isolate the nerve and to avoid iatrogenic injury. Once the terminal neuroma is found (see **Fig. 1**) and separated from surrounding tissues, it is excised completely with a knife until healthy-appearing axons are visualized. Depending on the location of the symptomatic neuroma, the free skeletal muscle graft can be obtained from a local muscle (eg, vastus lateralis after above-knee amputation or brachioradialis after transradial amputation). If access to the donor muscle can be obtained through the incision used to isolate the symptomatic neuroma, this should be attempted first; otherwise, a separate incision should be made over the desired donor muscle. The type of skeletal muscle (slow twitch or fast twitch) has not been shown to affect muscle graft reinnervation when reimplanted with a peripheral nerve, although surgeons should avoid using any muscle that could be advantageous for soft tissue padding with regard to prosthetic use.[88]

Regarding RPNI surgery for peripheral nerves involved during major limb amputation, free skeletal muscle grafts should be harvested from healthy muscle in the direction of fibers and ideally be 30 to 40 mm long, 15 to 20 mm wide, and 5 to 6 mm thick.[83] Because the devascularized skeletal muscle graft must undergo neovascularization, care must be taken to ensure that the muscle grafts are not too thick because this can affect survivability of the muscle graft during the imbibition phase.[60,68,89] Muscle grafts that are too large will undergo central necrosis and this deters from optimal reinnervation. After harvesting the free muscle graft, the peripheral nerve end is implanted parallel to the direction of the fibers and the epineurium is secured to the free muscle graft using a nonabsorbable monofilament suture such as 6-0 nylon. In addition, the edges of the free muscle graft are wrapped around the nerve and secured with sutures to create a cylindrical structure (see **Fig. 1**). The RPNI is then placed in a tension-free manner as far away from the surgical incision as possible and to avoid locating the RPNI near the weight-bearing surfaces of the residual limb. For large-caliber nerves, such as the sciatic nerve, intraneural dissection is recommended to separate the nerve into component fascicles to create several distinct RPNIs (see **Fig. 1**). Doing so optimizes the ratios of regenerating axons and denervated muscle fibers within the free graft. If component fascicular separation is not performed, 1 of 2 unfavorable outcomes is expected to occur: (1) there are too many regenerating axons in the peripheral nerve for the free muscle graft and those axons that do not undergo synaptogenesis will form a neuroma within the RPNI; (2) an exceedingly large free muscle graft is used for the peripheral nerve and it undergoes central necrosis during the process of revascularization, leading to suboptimal reinnervation and neuroma formation within the RPNI. Following RPNI surgery, the surgical incision (and additional donor site incision, if used) is closed in a layered fashion and a compression dressing used for several weeks.

RPNIs are also used to prevent neuroma formation in a prophylactic manner at the time of amputation surgery (**Fig. 3**). When amputation is not performed for tumor or ischemic indications, the free skeletal muscle grafts can readily be obtained from the amputation limb. The intended benefit of prophylactic RPNI surgery is to minimize postoperative residual limb pain, the experience of phantom limb pain, and the peripherally mediated mechanisms that lead to central sensitization and chronic pain. Depending on the level of the amputation, all major peripheral nerves should be considered for RPNI surgery. For instance, in a below-knee amputation, RPNI surgery can readily be performed for the tibial, deep peroneal, superficial peroneal, sural, and saphenous nerves.

Outcomes

Success from using RPNI surgery to both treat and prevent postamputation pain has resulted in widespread adoption of this treatment strategy across several surgical specialties at our institution. Favorable outcomes have been echoed by emerging clinical data. In a retrospective study comprising 16 patients and 17 residual limbs where 46 RPNIs were performed for postamputation neuroma pain treatment, there were significant reductions in neuroma pain scores and phantom pain scores at an average of 7.5 months postoperatively.[90] Mean neuroma pain score

reduced 71% from 8.7 preoperatively to 2.5 postoperatively ($P<.001$), and mean phantom pain score reduced 53% from 8.0 preoperatively to 3.8 postoperatively ($P = .009$). Importantly, most patients in this study reported reduction in pain medication use postoperatively as well as significant improvements in pain interference scores (a metric for how much an individual's pain experience interferes with life and daily activities).

Prophylactic RPNI surgery is also associated with favorable outcomes. In a retrospective review with matched controls, 0 of 45 patients who underwent RPNI at the time of primary amputation developed symptomatic neuromas after major limb amputation compared with 6 of 45 patients (13.3%) who did not undergo RPNI at the time of amputation ($P = .026$).[91] There was also a significant difference ($P<.0001$) in the incidence of phantom limb pain postoperatively; only 23 RPNI patients (51.1%) developed phantom limb pain compared with 41 control patients (91.1%). The mean follow-up in this study was 357 days in the RPNI group and 358 days in the control group. The study also emphasized that the complication rate in the prophylactic RPNI group was not any greater than in the control group despite RPNI surgery adding about an hour to the total operative time.

Complications

In general, complications following RPNI surgery are well tolerated by patients and do not detract from satisfaction regarding the surgical outcome. In the aforementioned study where 46 RPNIs were implanted into 16 patients, 75% of patients were satisfied or highly satisfied with pain relief, and 94% reported they would undergo surgery again if given the option.[90] Complications that have been reported after RPNI surgery include delayed wound healing, hematoma, and surgical site infections.[90] Clinically, almost all cases with delayed wound healing can be managed with local wound care and rarely require operative intervention.

Occasionally, successful treatment of 1 symptomatic neuroma unmasks a previously unidentified additional neuroma within the residual limb, necessitating further surgery. Formation of a neuroma within the RPNI muscle graft is possible and can result in persistent symptoms; to reduce the risk of recurrent neuroma formation, every effort should be focused on maximizing reinnervation (eg, performing fascicular RPNIs for nerves of larger caliber). Based on the available clinical data, RPNI surgery can be safely performed in patients with comorbidities such as peripheral vascular disease, diabetes, positive smoking status, osteomyelitis, coagulopathy, and trauma.

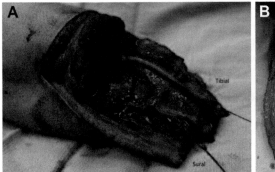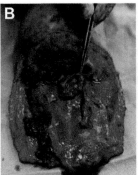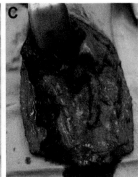

Fig. 3. Prophylactic creation of RPNIs in the lower extremity. (*A*) Identification of the tibial nerve and sural nerve after below-knee-amputation. (*B*) After RPNIs are performed of the tibial and sural nerve, (*C*) they are positioned appropriately to avoid compression by the tibia and to avoid external compression, such as from use of a prosthetic device. (*From* Santosa KB, Oliver JD, Cederna PS, Kung TA. Regenerative Peripheral Nerve Interfaces for Prevention and Management of Neuromas. Clin Plast Surg. 2020;47(2):311-321.)

Postoperative Recovery and Prosthetic Rehabilitation

RPNI surgery does not seem to delay prosthetic rehabilitation. Postoperative compression garments or wraps are used to help minimize postoperative edema. Soft tissue healing is typically complete in 4 to 6 weeks, whereas any areas of delayed wound healing are usually managed with local wound care. In these cases, complete healing typically occurs after an additional 3 to 4 weeks. Typically, 2 to 3 months after surgery when soft tissue healing has occurred, postoperative edema resolved, and pain control attained, patients are able to meet with a physiatrist and prosthetist to start prosthetic rehabilitation.

When performed prophylactically in conjunction with major limb amputation, RPNI surgery does not significantly prolong patient recovery and healing time.[91] In our clinical experience, many patients report that RPNI surgery has facilitated prosthetic rehabilitation and that they are able to wear a functional prosthetic limb for longer periods of time. Studies have shown that improved comfort associated with prosthetic devices results in improvements with prosthetic compliance and, presumably, improved participation in rehabilitation.[92–94] Therefore, prophylactic RPNIs may play a crucial role in maintaining prosthetic device use and rehabilitation among patients with new amputations.

Use of Regenerative Peripheral Nerve Interfaces in Other Clinical Applications and Future Directions

In addition to its role in reducing postamputation pain, ongoing investigation is examining the potential for the RPNI to serve as a novel neuroprosthetic interface. RPNIs can harness motor control signals from transected peripheral nerves with high signal-to-noise ratios and these can be used to generate complex movements of an artificial limb. Furthermore, emerging evidence has shown that RPNIs have the potential to facilitate sensory feedback through afferent stimulation.[95,96] These exciting preliminary data suggest that RPNI surgery may be a revolutionary surgical technique that can offer 3 important goals of amputation rehabilitation: (1) mitigation of postamputation pain, (2) intuitive prosthetic control, and (3) meaningful sensory feedback.

Furthermore, given the physiologic basis of the RPNI using a free muscle graft, a transected sensory nerve that would normally innervate skin may be able to reinnervate a free dermal graft. Using this approach, variations of the RPNI known as dermal sensory peripheral nerve interfaces have been tested successfully in animal models to transduce sensory nerve action potentials.[96] Investigations are also being performed on composite RPNIs (C-RPNIs) that are designed to simultaneously capture efferent motor and afferent sensory signals.[97] The C-RPNI comprises a free dermal and muscle graft secured around a target mixed sensorimotor nerve. Together, these early findings show great promise for the potential of peripheral nerve interfaces in advancing patient experiences during prosthetic rehabilitation.

Other clinical applications for RPNIs could be in the setting of addressing neuropathic pain seen after abdominal surgery (eg, inguinal hernia repair), obstetric and gynecologic surgery (eg, cesarean section and hysterectomy), and head and neck surgery (eg, parotidectomy).[98–100] In these cases, various injured nerves, such as the ilioinguinal, iliohypogastric, genitofemoral, and greater auricular, have been treated by different passive techniques with variable success. By using RPNIs, a major limitation of current passive techniques is overcome by providing injured peripheral nerves distal targets for regenerating axons, which in turn minimizes aberrant axonal growth and sprouting that would lead to symptomatic neuroma formation and patient discomfort. Further studies investigating the efficacy of RPNIs in these settings are currently underway.

SUMMARY

The RPNI represents a paradigm shift in the approach to treating neuroma pain because it focuses on providing reinnervation targets for regenerating peripheral nerves. RPNI surgery has shown promise in early clinical studies and is a safe, physiologic, and straightforward surgical technique to treat and prevent neuroma pain and phantom limb pain. Ongoing investigational trials will help elucidate the critical role of RPNI surgery in a variety of clinical scenarios.

CLINICS CARE POINTS

- Regenerative Peripheral Nerve Interfaces (RPNIs) can be used to treat and prevent neuromas and neuroma pain.
- RPNIs have been used to mitigate neuroma pain and phantom pain in the upper and lower extremity after amputation.
- When RPNI surgery is performed on large caliber nerves, e.g. sciatic, intraneural dissection is recommended to separate the nerve into component fascicles to create individual RPNIs. This optimizes ratio of regenerating axons to denervated muscle fibers within the free graft.
- Muscle grafts for RPNI surgery should be harvested from healthy muscle with careful attention given to the dimensions of the graft. Survivability of muscle grafts that are thicker than 5-6 mm may be affected during the imbibition phase. Similarly, muscle grafts that are too large may undergo central necrosis and this deters from optimal reinnervation.
- In general, complications following RPNI surgery are well-tolerated by patients and do not detract from satisfaction regarding the surgical outcome. Furthermore, RPNI surgery does not appear to delay prosthetic rehabilitation or prolong patient recovery.

DISCLOSURE

The authors have no commercial or financial conflicts of interest and no funding sources for the work presented in this article.

REFERENCES

1. Lee MG, Bahman. Nerves and nerve injuries, chapter 7 - postoperative neuromasVol 2. Waltham (MA): Elsevier; 2015. Pain, Treatment, Injury, Disease and Future Directions.
2. Zabaglo M, Dreyer MA. Neuroma. Treasure Island (FL): StatPearls; 2020.
3. Sayan NB, Ucok C. Asymptomatic traumatic neuroma after mandibular sagittal split osteotomy: a case report. J Oral Maxillofac Surg 2002;60(1): 111–2.
4. Lee EJ, Calcaterra TC, Zuckerbraun L. Traumatic neuromas of the head and neck. Ear Nose Throat J 1998;77(8):670–4, 676.
5. Bi A, Park E, Dumanian GA. Treatment of Painful Nerves in the Abdominal Wall Using Processed Nerve Allografts. Plast Reconstr Surg Glob Open 2018;6(3):e1670.
6. Li Q, Gao EL, Yang YL, et al. Traumatic neuroma in a patient with breast cancer after mastectomy: a case report and review of the literature. World J Surg Oncol 2012;10:35.
7. Souza JM, Purnell CA, Cheesborough JE, et al. Treatment of Foot and Ankle Neuroma Pain With Processed Nerve Allografts. Foot Ankle Int 2016; 37(10):1098–105.
8. Hsu E, Cohen SP. Postamputation pain: epidemiology, mechanisms, and treatment. J Pain Res 2013;6:121–36.
9. Geraghty TJ, Jones LE. Painful neuromata following upper limb amputation. Prosthet Orthot Int 1996;20(3):176–81.
10. Soroush M, Modirian E, Soroush M, et al. Neuroma in bilateral upper limb amputation. Orthopedics 2008;31(12). https://doi.org/10.3928/01477447-20081201-26.
11. Ehde DM, Czerniecki JM, Smith DG, et al. Chronic phantom sensations, phantom pain, residual limb pain, and other regional pain after lower limb amputation. Arch Phys Med Rehabil 2000;81(8): 1039–44.
12. Jensen TS, Krebs B, Nielsen J, et al. Immediate and long-term phantom limb pain in amputees: incidence, clinical characteristics and relationship to pre-amputation limb pain. Pain 1985;21(3): 267–78.
13. Kuffler DP. Origins of Phantom Limb Pain. Mol Neurobiol 2018;55(1):60–9.
14. Kaur A, Guan Y. Phantom limb pain: A literature review. Chin J Traumatol 2018;21(6):366–8.

15. Aternali A, Katz J. Recent advances in understanding and managing phantom limb pain. F1000Res 2019;8. https://doi.org/10.12688/f1000research. 19355.1.

16. Economides JM, DeFazio MV, Attinger CE, et al. Prevention of painful neuroma and phantom limb pain after transfemoral amputations through concomitant nerve coaptation and collagen nerve wrapping. Neurosurgery 2016;79(3): 508–13.

17. Nikolajsen L. Postamputation pain: studies on mechanisms. Dan Med J 2012;59(10):B4527.

18. Becher S, Smith M, Ziran B. Orthopaedic trauma patients and depression: a prospective cohort. J Orthop Trauma 2014;28(10):e242–6.

19. Bhutani S, Bhutani J, Chhabra A, et al. Living with Amputation: Anxiety and Depression Correlates. J Clin Diagn Res 2016;10(9):RC09–12.

20. Humble SR, Dalton AJ, Li L. A systematic review of therapeutic interventions to reduce acute and chronic post-surgical pain after amputation, thoracotomy or mastectomy. Eur J Pain 2015;19(4): 451–65.

21. Gaudet AD, Popovich PG, Ramer MS. Wallerian degeneration: gaining perspective on inflammatory events after peripheral nerve injury. J Neuroinflammation 2011;8:110.

22. Menorca RM, Fussell TS, Elfar JC. Nerve physiology: mechanisms of injury and recovery. Hand Clin 2013;29(3):317–30.

23. Oliveira KMC, Pindur L, Han Z, et al. Time course of traumatic neuroma development. PLoS One 2018; 13(7):e0200548.

24. Wood MD, Mackinnon SE. Pathways regulating modality-specific axonal regeneration in peripheral nerve. Exp Neurol 2015;265:171–5.

25. Foltan R, Klima K, Spackova J, et al. Mechanism of traumatic neuroma development. Med Hypotheses 2008;71(4):572–6.

26. Stokvis A, van der Avoort DJ, van Neck JW, et al. Surgical management of neuroma pain: a prospective follow-up study. Pain 2010;151(3):862–9.

27. Curtin C, Carroll I. Cutaneous neuroma physiology and its relationship to chronic pain. J Hand Surg Am 2009;34(7):1334–6.

28. Hains BC, Klein JP, Saab CY, et al. Upregulation of sodium channel Nav1.3 and functional involvement in neuronal hyperexcitability associated with central neuropathic pain after spinal cord injury. J Neurosci 2003;23(26):8881–92.

29. Watson J, Gonzalez M, Romero A, et al. Neuromas of the hand and upper extremity. J Hand Surg Am 2010;35(3):499–510.

30. Stokvis A, Ruijs AC, van Neck JW, et al. Cold intolerance in surgically treated neuroma patients: a prospective follow-up study. J Hand Surg Am 2009;34(9):1689–95.

31. Sehirlioglu A, Ozturk C, Yazicioglu K, et al. Painful neuroma requiring surgical excision after lower limb amputation caused by landmine explosions. Int Orthop 2009;33(2):533–6.

32. Nguyen JT, Buchanan IA, Patel PP, et al. Intercostal neuroma as a source of pain after aesthetic and reconstructive breast implant surgery. J Plast Reconstr Aesthet Surg 2012;65(9):1199–203.

33. Donnal JF, Blinder RA, Coblentz CL, et al. MR imaging of stump neuroma. J Comput Assist Tomogr 1990;14(4):656–7.

34. Singson RD, Feldman F, Slipman CW, et al. Postamputation neuromas and other symptomatic stump abnormalities: detection with CT. Radiology 1987;162(3):743–5.

35. Henrot P, Stines J, Walter F, et al. Imaging of the painful lower limb stump. Radiographics 2000; 20(Spec No):S219–35.

36. Singson RD, Feldman F, Staron R, et al. MRI of postamputation neuromas. Skeletal Radiol 1990; 19(4):259–62.

37. Provost N, Bonaldi VM, Sarazin L, et al. Amputation stump neuroma: ultrasound features. J Clin Ultrasound 1997;25(2):85–9.

38. Buchheit T, Van de Ven T, Hsia HL, et al. Pain phenotypes and associated clinical risk factors following traumatic amputation: results from veterans integrated pain evaluation research (VIPER). Pain Med 2016;17(1):149–61.

39. Penna A, Konstantatos AH, Cranwell W, et al. Incidence and associations of painful neuroma in a contemporary cohort of lower-limb amputees. ANZ J Surg 2018;88(5):491–6.

40. Latremoliere A, Woolf CJ. Central sensitization: a generator of pain hypersensitivity by central neural plasticity. J Pain 2009;10(9):895–926.

41. Dydyk AMGA. Central pain syndrome. StatPearls. Treasure Island (FL): StatPearls Publishing; 2020. Available at: https://www.ncbi.nlm.nih. gov/books/NBK553027/. Accessed February 1, 2021.

42. Schwartzman RJ, Grothusen J, Kiefer TR, et al. Neuropathic central pain: epidemiology, etiology, and treatment options. Arch Neurol 2001;58(10): 1547–50.

43. Woolf CJ. A new strategy for the treatment of inflammatory pain. Prevention or elimination of central sensitization. Drugs 1994;47(Suppl 5):1–9 [discussion: 46–7].

44. Campbell JN, Meyer RA. Mechanisms of neuropathic pain. Neuron 2006;52(1):77–92.

45. Stokvis A, Coert JH, van Neck JW. Insufficient pain relief after surgical neuroma treatment: Prognostic factors and central sensitisation. J Plast Reconstr Aesthet Surg 2010;63(9):1538–43.

46. Ducic I, Mesbahi AN, Attinger CE, et al. The role of peripheral nerve surgery in the treatment of chronic

pain associated with amputation stumps. Plast Reconstr Surg 2008;121(3):908–14 [discussion: 915–7].

47. Dellon AL, Mackinnon SE. Treatment of the painful neuroma by neuroma resection and muscle implantation. Plast Reconstr Surg 1986;77(3):427–38.

48. Burchiel KJ, Johans TJ, Ochoa J. The surgical treatment of painful traumatic neuromas. J Neurosurg 1993;78(5):714–9.

49. Robbins TH. Nerve capping in the treatment of troublesome terminal neuromata. Br J Plast Surg 1986;39(2):239–40.

50. Pet MA, Ko JH, Friedly JL, et al. Does targeted nerve implantation reduce neuroma pain in amputees? Clin Orthop Relat Res 2014;472(10):2991–3001.

51. Zhang X, Xu Y, Zhou J, et al. Ultrasound-guided alcohol neurolysis and radiofrequency ablation of painful stump neuroma: effective treatments for post-amputation pain. J Pain Res 2017;10:295–302.

52. Hung YH, Wu CH, Ozcakar L, et al. Ultrasound-Guided Steroid Injections for Two Painful Neuromas in the Stump of a Below-Elbow Amputee. Am J Phys Med Rehabil 2016;95(5):e73–4.

53. Soin A, Fang ZP, Velasco J. Peripheral Neuromodulation to Treat Postamputation Pain. Prog Neurol Surg 2015;29:158–67.

54. Dahl E, Cohen SP. Perineural injection of etanercept as a treatment for postamputation pain. Clin J Pain 2008;24(2):172–5.

55. Salminger S, Sturma A, Roche AD, et al. Outcomes, challenges and pitfalls after targeted muscle reinnervation in high level amputees. Is it worth the effort? Plast Reconstr Surg 2019;144(6):1037e–43e.

56. Eberlin KR, Ducic I. Surgical algorithm for neuroma management: a changing treatment paradigm. Plast Reconstr Surg Glob Open 2018;6(10):e1952.

57. Poppler LH, Parikh RP, Bichanich MJ, et al. Surgical interventions for the treatment of painful neuroma: a comparative meta-analysis. Pain 2018;159(2):214–23.

58. Domeshek LF, Krauss EM, Snyder-Warwick AK, et al. Surgical treatment of neuromas improves patient-reported pain, depression, and quality of life. Plast Reconstr Surg 2017;139(2):407–18.

59. Dumanian GA, Potter BK, Mioton LM, et al. Targeted muscle reinnervation treats neuroma and phantom pain in major limb amputees: a randomized clinical trial. Ann Surg 2019;270(2):238–46.

60. Ives GC, Kung TA, Nghiem BT, et al. Current state of the surgical treatment of terminal neuromas. Neurosurgery 2018;83(3):354–64.

61. Melanie G, Urbanchek BW, Baghmanli Z, et al. Cederna. Long-Term Stability of Regenerative Peripheral Nerve Interfaces (RPNI). Plast Reconstr Surg 2011;128(Supplement 4S):88–9.

62. Langhals NB, Woo SL, Moon JD, et al. Electrically stimulated signals from a long-term Regenerative Peripheral Nerve Interface. Conf Proc IEEE Eng Med Biol Soc 2014;2014:1989–92.

63. Kung TA, Bueno RA, Alkhalefah GK, et al. Innovations in prosthetic interfaces for the upper extremity. Plast Reconstr Surg 2013;132(6):1515–23.

64. Vu PP, Vaskov AK, Irwin ZT, et al. A regenerative peripheral nerve interface allows real-time control of an artificial hand in upper limb amputees. Sci Transl Med 2020;12(533):eaay2857.

65. Kung TA, Langhals NB, Martin DC, et al. Regenerative peripheral nerve interface viability and signal transduction with an implanted electrode. Plast Reconstr Surg 2014;133(6):1380–94.

66. Irwin ZT, Schroeder KE, Vu PP, et al. Chronic recording of hand prosthesis control signals via a regenerative peripheral nerve interface in a rhesus macaque. J Neural Eng 2016;13(4):046007.

67. Woo SL, Urbanchek MG, Cederna PS, et al. Revisiting nonvascularized partial muscle grafts: a novel use for prosthetic control. Plast Reconstr Surg 2014;134(2):344e–6e.

68. Hu Y, VanBelkum AL, Sando IC, et al. Muscle graft volume implanted in regenerative peripheral nerve interfaces influences electrical signal transduction. Waikoloa, Hawaii: American Association for Hand Surgery; 2017. p. 2017.

69. Carlson BM, Faulkner JA. The regeneration of skeletal muscle fibers following injury: a review. Med Sci Sports Exerc 1983;15(3):187–98.

70. Chappell AG, Jordan SW, Dumanian GA. Targeted Muscle Reinnervation for Treatment of Neuropathic Pain. Clin Plast Surg 2020;47(2):285–93.

71. Kuiken TA, Li G, Lock BA, et al. Targeted muscle reinnervation for real-time myoelectric control of multifunction artificial arms. JAMA 2009;301(6):619–28.

72. Kuiken TA, Dumanian GA, Lipschutz RD, et al. The use of targeted muscle reinnervation for improved myoelectric prosthesis control in a bilateral shoulder disarticulation amputee. Prosthet Orthot Int 2004;28(3):245–53.

73. Hijjawi JB, Kuiken TA, Lipschutz RD, et al. Improved myoelectric prosthesis control accomplished using multiple nerve transfers. Plast Reconstr Surg 2006;118(7):1573–8.

74. Kuiken TA, Miller LA, Lipschutz RD, et al. Targeted reinnervation for enhanced prosthetic arm function in a woman with a proximal amputation: a case study. Lancet 2007;369(9559):371–80.

75. O'Shaughnessy KD, Dumanian GA, Lipschutz RD, et al. Targeted reinnervation to improve prosthesis control in transhumeral amputees. A report of

three cases. J Bone Joint Surg Am 2008;90(2): 393–400.

76. Valerio IL, Dumanian GA, Jordan SW, et al. Preemptive treatment of phantom and residual limb pain with targeted muscle reinnervation at the time of major limb amputation. J Am Coll Surg 2019;228(3):217–26.

77. Kim PS, Ko J, O'Shaughnessy KK, et al. Novel model for end-neuroma formation in the amputated rabbit forelimb. J Brachial Plex Peripher Nerve Inj 2010;5:6.

78. Kim PS, Ko JH, O'Shaughnessy KK, et al. The effects of targeted muscle reinnervation on neuromas in a rabbit rectus abdominis flap model. J Hand Surg Am 2012;37(8):1609–16.

79. Souza JM, Cheesborough JE, Ko JH, et al. Targeted muscle reinnervation: a novel approach to postamputation neuroma pain. Clin Orthop Relat Res 2014;472(10):2984–90.

80. Subedi B, Grossberg GT. Phantom limb pain: mechanisms and treatment approaches. Pain Res Treat 2011;2011:864605.

81. Gart MS, Souza JM, Dumanian GA. Targeted muscle reinnervation in the upper extremity amputee: a technical roadmap. J Hand Surg Am 2015;40(9): 1877–88.

82. Mavrogenis AF, Pavlakis K, Stamatoukou A, et al. Current treatment concepts for neuromas-in-continuity. Injury 2008;39(Suppl 3):S43–8.

83. Kubiak CA, Kemp SWP, Cederna PS. Regenerative peripheral nerve interface for management of postamputation neuroma. JAMA Surg 2018;153(7): 681–2.

84. Neil M. Pain after amputation. BJA Educ 2016; 16(3):107–12.

85. Potter BK, Forsberg JA, Davis TA, et al. Heterotopic ossification following combat-related trauma. J Bone Joint Surg Am volume 2010;92(Suppl 2): 74–89.

86. Eisenstein N, Stapley S, Grover L. Post-traumatic heterotopic ossification: an old problem in need of new solutions. J Orthop Res 2018;36(4):1061–8.

87. Edwards DS, Clasper JC. Heterotopic ossification: a systematic review. J R Army Med Corps 2015; 161(4):315–21.

88. Woo SLU, Melanie G, Zheng Xin, et al. Partial Skeletal Muscle Grafts for Prosthetic Control. Plast Reconstr Surg 2014;134(4S-1):55–6.

89. White TP, Devor ST. Skeletal muscle regeneration and plasticity of grafts. Exerc Sport Sci Rev 1993; 21:263–95.

90. Woo SL, Kung TA, Brown DL, et al. Regenerative peripheral nerve interfaces for the treatment of postamputation neuroma pain: a pilot study. Plast Reconstr Surg Glob Open 2016;4(12):e1038.

91. Kubiak CA, Kemp SWP, Cederna PS, et al. Prophylactic Regenerative Peripheral Nerve Interfaces to Prevent Postamputation Pain. Plast Reconstr Surg 2019;144(3):421e–30e.

92. Noah Rosenblatt TE, Fergus R, Bauer A, et al. Effects of vacuum-assisted socket suspension on energetic costs of walking, functional mobility, and prosthesis-related quality of life. J Prosthetics Orthotics 2017;29(2):65–72.

93. Astrom I, Stenstrom A. Effect on gait and socket comfort in unilateral trans-tibial amputees after exchange to a polyurethane concept. Prosthet Orthot Int 2004;28(1):28–36.

94. Baars EC, Geertzen JH. Literature review of the possible advantages of silicon liner socket use in trans-tibial prostheses. Prosthet Orthot Int 2005; 29(1):27–37.

95. Vu P, Lu C, Vaskov A, et al. Restoration of proprioceptive and cutaneous sensation using Regenerative Peripheral Nerve Interfaces (RPNIs) in humans with upper-limb amputations. Plast Reconstr Surg Glob Open 2020;8(4 Suppl):65.

96. Sando ICG, Gregory J, Ursu DC, et al. Dermal-Based Peripheral Nerve Interface for Transduction of Sensory Feedback. Plast Reconstr Surg 2015; 136(4S):19–20.

97. Svientek SR, Ursu DC, Cederna PS, et al. Fabrication of the Composite Regenerative Peripheral Nerve Interface (C-RPNI) in the Adult Rat. J Vis Exp 2020;(156). https://doi.org/10.3791/60841.

98. Gangopadhyay N, Pothula A, Yao A, et al. Retroperitoneal Approach for Ilioinguinal, Iliohypogastric, and Genitofemoral Neurectomies in the Treatment of Refractory Groin Pain After Inguinal Hernia Repair. Ann Plast Surg 2020;84(4):431–5.

99. de Ru JA, Thomeer H, Tijink BM, et al. Neurocap use for the treatment of iatrogenic neuropathic pain: preliminary operative results in 3 patients. Ear Nose Throat J 2020. https://doi.org/10.1177/0145561320912048. 145561320912048.

100. Ducic I, Moxley M, Al-Attar A. Algorithm for treatment of postoperative incisional groin pain after cesarean delivery or hysterectomy. Obstet Gynecol 2006;108(1):27–31.

Nerve Interface Strategies for Neuroma Management and Prevention
A Conceptual Approach Guided by Institutional Experience

Benjamin W. Hoyt, MD[a], Benjamin K. Potter, MD[a], Jason M. Souza, MD[b,*]

KEYWORDS

- Targeted muscular reinnervation • Regenerative peripheral nerve interface • Amputation
- Nerve interface strategy

KEY POINTS

- For targeted muscle reinnervation and regenerative peripheral nerve interface, denervation is critical to providing a neurotropic signal necessary for coordinated nerve regeneration. In the absence of neurotropic support, proximal segment axons form disorganized sprouts.
- Nerve interface strategies can be varied or combined for the needs of the clinical situation so long as this underlying concept is maintained.
- Neuroma prevention strategies should be formulated based on the predictable pattern of neuroma development after amputation rather than increase morbidity by addressing every cut peripheral nerve.

INTRODUCTION

Increased sophistication of amputation techniques and improved prosthetic capabilities have fostered a dramatic shift in patient and surgeon attitudes toward amputation, resulting in renewed interest in amputation surgery. Once considered the unfortunate consequence of failed reconstructive efforts, amputation is increasingly being viewed as a functionally restorative procedure.[1,2] Unfortunately, the potential benefits of amputation, when weighed against a painful or dysfunctional "salvaged" limb, have often been obscured by the high rates of debilitating neuroma or phantom limb pain associated with conventional amputation.[3,4] Recently, nerve interface procedures,

such as targeted muscle reinnervation (TMR) and the regenerative peripheral nerve interface (RPNI), have provided effective means to treat or prevent neuromata and phantom limb pain, thus opening the door to further innovation in amputation surgery.

TMR and RPNI reflect relatively recent innovations in the surgical management of neuromas and rehabilitation with myoelectric prostheses. Both techniques were first described for improving terminal device control in major upper-extremity amputation, using different sources of expendable muscle or muscle grafts, respectively, to serve as biologic amplifiers of the donor nerves' native signals. TMR has been increasingly and successfully used in upper-extremity amputees for this purpose

Funding Sources: Funding for submission was provided by the USU-Walter Reed Department of Surgery.
[a] USU-Walter Reed Department of Surgery, Walter Reed National Military Medical Center, Uniformed Services University, 8901 Wisconsin Avenue, Bethesda, MD 20814, USA; [b] Peripheral Nerve Program, USU-Walter Reed Department of Surgery, Walter Reed National Military Medical Center, Uniformed Services University, 8901 Wisconsin Avenue, Bethesda, MD 20814, USA
* Corresponding author.
E-mail address: jasonmsouza@gmail.com

Hand Clin 37 (2021) 373–382
https://doi.org/10.1016/j.hcl.2021.05.004
0749-0712/21/Published by Elsevier Inc.

for nearly 2 decades, and the technique's control benefits can be successfully harnessed with commercially available components using either direct control (1 muscle, 1 prosthetic function) and advanced pattern recognition (permitting additional degrees of freedom) techniques. RPNI has also been successful to this end but requires either implanted myoelectric sensors/transmitters or transcutaneous wires to harness the prosthetic control potential. Subsequently, both TMR and RPNI were incidentally found to prevent the formation or recurrence of symptomatic neuromata in major and minor extremity amputees when compared with conventional nerve interventions.[5–7]

These interventions represent a paradigm shift in the management of amputation-related nerve pain. Rather than attempt to prevent nerve regeneration through purposeful nerve destruction or containment, or through moving the inevitable neuroma to a less symptomatic location, TMR and RPNI provide reliable methods for fostering coordinated regeneration of transected mixed motor and sensory nerves. Application of these techniques has generated favorable pain outcomes in increasingly larger and more scientifically robust clinical studies. A randomized controlled trial for treatment of pain with delayed TMR versus neurectomy and nerve burial in local innervated muscle demonstrated improvements in phantom and residual limb pain, although the latter did not reach significance.[1] In a case series, RPNI also demonstrated significant improvements in both phantom and neuroma pain at 3 to 15 months after surgery.[8]

A growing body of evidence further suggests that both these strategies may be more effective when used prophylactically at the time of the initial amputation, although this has not yet been compared directly. Kubiak and colleagues[9] performed a case-control series comparing prophylactic RPNI at the time of amputation and described no reported neuroma pain and reduced phantom limb pain compared with standard management. Comparing their experience with a large general amputee population, Valerio and colleagues[10] reported decreased phantom and residual limb pain and improved patient-reported outcomes when TMR was performed at the time of amputation. It is unclear whether these comparatively better results may be due to pain potentiation effects,[11,12] neuronal signal amplification pathways or retrograde axonal sprouting after delayed intervention,[13] a temporal decline in neuronal regenerative capacity,[14] or another as yet unknown mechanism.

Despite limited available outcomes data and as yet poorly understood mechanisms of putative

efficacy, there has been tremendous interest in the use of these techniques in the primary amputation setting. Prophylactic use of nerve interface strategies is largely motivated by experience with treatment-refractory phantom limb pain, and the belief that prevention, if achievable, will be more effective than any available management strategy. At some institutions, these techniques have already become a standard component of extremity amputation, similar to a well-performed myodesis or posterior myocutaneous flap for transtibial coverage. Herein, we aim to describe the rationale behind our use of TMR and RPNI in isolation, concurrently, or with hybrid modifications, as well as report our experience with these techniques based on the level and amputation setting.

CONCEPTUAL FRAMEWORK

The best way to treat or prevent neuroma formation and subsequent pain is to provide the necessary elements to foster coordinated and physiologic nerve regeneration. Conceptually, this means providing the regenerating proximal nerve with a distal target, neurotrophic signals, and a pathway or conduit across which to regenerate (**Fig. 1**). In the intact traumatically injured extremity, where transected nerves may form traumatic neuromas or neuromas-in-continuity, this is best accomplished by repairing or reconstructing the nerve when possible.[15] Even in the absence of functional recovery, painful neuroma formation after repair or reconstruction is uncommon.[16] However, this relies on the presence of a native distal nerve segment and end organ target, which is by definition absent following amputation. These critical components for physiologic nerve regeneration can be restored via replantation or vascularized composite tissue transplantation, but these are impractical solutions in many clinical scenarios. However, they can be viewed conceptually as the gold standard against which other nerve management strategies should be weighed.

By providing a recipient nerve, a denervated muscle target, and neurotrophic signals to guide regeneration, TMR best approximates the nerve regeneration environment offered by replantation/transplantation. Giving the nerve "somewhere to go and something to do" fosters a regenerative process that more closely mimics a primary nerve repair than the chaotic sprouting that drives neuroma formation.[7] In its purest form, TMR refers to identification and transection of a motor nerve branch to an expendable muscle or muscle segment in the region of a transected mixed motor or sensory nerve. The transected mixed or sensory nerve is then mobilized and coaptated to the

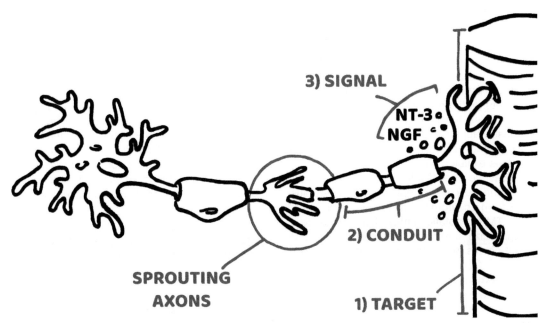

3) SIGNAL

NT-3
NGF

2) CONDUIT

**SPROUTING
AXONS**

1) TARGET

Fig. 1. Conceptual framework for nerve regeneration. Following nerve injury, optimal nerve regeneration occurs in the presence of a denervated end organ target (1), a nerve conduit through which to guide sprouting axons (2), and neurotrophic signals that coordinate the process of regeneration (3).

recipient motor nerve branch in end-to-end fashion, whereas the proximal portion of the transected motor branch is left to form a small, asymptomatic neuroma. More than a half-century of muscle flap-based reconstructions have demonstrated motor nerve neuroma formation to be clinically irrelevant.

In lieu of a recipient nerve and vascularly intact muscle segment, RPNI uses a devascularized muscle graft as a reinnervation target. The transected nerve can be left intact or separated into fascicle groups and then wrapped in a muscle graft with dimensions of approximately 1 × 3 cm. The 3-cm length is thought to be necessary to ensure inclusion of sufficient myomeres and neuromuscular junctions. The technique is not dependent on identification of a recipient motor nerve nor is it constrained by the need to maintain perfusion to the muscle target. The graft is subsequently revascularized by the wound bed peripherally, and the vasa nervorum of the buried nerve centrally. The regenerating nerve is thus provided a denervated target for regeneration that offers the sprouting axons "something to do." However, conventional RPNI lacks the nerve conduit provided by TMR's recipient motor nerve. The clinical significance of this difference is unknown, but in this way, RPNI is less comparable to the aforementioned conceptual gold standard.

Importantly, both TMR and RPNI offer denervated targets for regeneration. Denervation is critical to providing the third component necessary for coordinated nerve regeneration: a neurotrophic signal.[17] Cell signaling studies have demonstrated that brain-derived neurotrophic factor (BDNF) expression is upregulated by denervated muscles and returns to normal levels after reinnervation.[18] Continuous BDNF release has been shown to decrease neuropathic pain in rodent models.[19] Insufficient neurotropic support, either through surplus axonal transfer or through inadequate innervation, yields neuroma formation. Denervation of the muscle target is the key quality that differentiates TMR and RPNI from the muscle-burying technique popularized by Dellon and MacKinnon.[20] Whereas muscle buying provides padding and an improved microenvironment for the unavoidably recurrent neuroma, it does not provide the setting necessary for coordinated regeneration because the recipient muscle is already innervated.[17] In the absence of this critical neurotropic support, proximal segment axons form disorganized sprouts marked by increased counts of myelinated fibers[21] and a higher frequency of spontaneous depolarization.[22] Preclinical studies have demonstrated decreased nerve sprouting and near-normal myelinated fiber counts following targeted muscle innervation.[21] Although not compared directly, RPNI appears to yield similar histologic improvements as TMR with respect to neuronal size and maturational/morphologic effects on the target muscle tissue.[23]

Denervation of the muscle target is thought to be critical to minimizing the likelihood of neuroma recurrence, although the importance of target volume and vascularity is not yet known. Below a requisite volume, there may be inadequate motor endplates to provide a sufficient number of muscle fiber targets for the regenerating axons. Although target muscles have been shown to adapt to more closely approximate the structure and function of the donor nerve's native muscle, the muscle target does exhibit a finite innervation capacity.[17] In the absence of available neuromuscular junctions or sufficient neurotrophic support, surplus neurons form a neuroma at the nerve-muscle interface.[8,17] TMR coaptations may also experience a significant size mismatch between donor and recipient nerves, which has the potential to dilute neurotropic factors and permit axonal escape and neuroma formation at the coaptation site.[24,25] However, the clinical significance of this interface neuroma is unclear, as this phenomenon has been observed radiographically in patients who have experienced resolution of pain symptoms following TMR. The role of target vascularity is equally undecided. Larger graft sizes may not remain viable particularly in the setting of a traumatic or dysvascular wound bed.[26] Despite early revascularization and maturation within 1 to 4 months, RPNI is associated with muscle graft volumetric loss or central necrosis when larger grafts are applied without reconstitution of vascularity.[27] Some investigators preferentially divide large nerves to improve the axon-to-muscle graft volume ratio and avoid necessity for these large grafts.[8] Recently, a vascularized RPNI technique has been proposed to overcome this perceived weakness of the RPNI strategy. Small, locally sourced muscle flaps are developed based on perforating vessels and then sutured around the transected nerve.[25] Given the uncertain influence of target perfusion on neuroma recurrence, it is unclear whether potential improvements in pain outcomes will justify the added complexity of this approach.

Further technical refinement of all nerve interface strategies is hampered by a severely limited understanding of the means by which they provide pain relief. As a result, it is difficult to weigh the relative importance of muscle volume, vascularity, or neurotrophic content in order to determine the optimal nerve interface strategy. Positive histomorphometric data and favorable cortical remapping on functional imaging are held up as objective evidence of a beneficial effect, but they do little to offer insight into the underlying mechanism. Some investigators have theorized that the provision of a physiologic pathway for neuronal regeneration restores an afferent signaling pathway from muscle sensory receptors, effectively closing the afferent-efferent signaling loop.[1] The positive clinical outcomes reported with use of the agonist-antagonist myoneural interfaces technique rely on a similar restoration of proprioceptive pathways,[28] which are then augmented with RPNI for the distal, transected nerves. Alternatively, nerve interface strategies may yield decreased pain by limiting the concentration of dysregulated depolarizing ion channels at the axonal tip.[29,30] Furthermore, pain relief may simply result from cessation of an overactive regeneration process.[31]

CLINICAL STRATEGY: BALANCING BENEFITS, MORBIDITY, AND COMPLEXITY

To date, TMR and RPNI have not been directly compared in a rigorous research setting. All available reports of TMR and RPNI for neuroma treatment or prevention describe a single-nerve interface strategy, often applied universally across all mixed and major sensory nerves.[1,6,9,32,33] In the absence of comparative data or a mechanistic understanding of their effects, clinical application of these nerve interface strategies requires consideration of the practical advantages and disadvantages of each technique (**Table 1**). As opposed to rigidly adhering to a specific technique, we have used nerve interface strategies based on belief in the underlying concept. As such, we have used each technique in isolation or in combination or have used hybrid modifications where needed to best meet the needs of the clinical situation.

We currently use 4 different nerve interface techniques in our clinical practice (**Fig. 2**). Our preferred approach to TMR involves a nerve coaptation between the donor and recipient nerve performed as close as possible to the motor entry point into the muscle target. Presented with a significant size mismatch, a single small-caliber suture is used to centralize the recipient nerve relative to the larger donor nerve diameter. Epineurial-to-epimysial sutures are then used to recruit the nearby target muscle to encompass the entirety of the donor nerve. This technique achieves a similar aim to that recently reported by Valerio and colleagues,[25] decreasing axonal escape and neuroma-in-situ from insufficient distal targets by providing freshly denervated motor endplates to capture sprouting mismatched axons, although without the need to formally elevate a local muscle flap. Conventional RPNI is typically performed as originally described by Kubiak and colleagues,[33] with muscle graft

Table 1
Benefits, morbidity, and complexity of nerve intervention strategies

Nerve Intervention Strategy	Benefits	Morbidity/Issues
TMR	• Greater available supporting literature • Theoretically ideal regenerative environment • Similar complication rate compared with other interventions	• Greater muscle denervation and atrophy (implications unclear) • Greater need for surgical exposure and nerve mobilization • Increased technical complexity
RPNI	• Minimal technical requirements/feasible without microsurgical skills • Minimal need to mobilize nerve • Minimal harvest site morbidity (particularly if taken from amputated muscle) • Increased available targets • Avoids denervation atrophy	• Uncertain whether sufficient neuromuscular junctions available in harvested graft depending on size • Concern for viability/revascularization of graft in traumatic or dysvascular wound bed • Graft size limitations
"In situ" vascularized RPNI (vRPNI)	• No revascularization of target required • Potentially unlimited muscle graft size • No additional dissection or muscle graft harvest required	• Requires a proximally denervated target through concurrent TMR procedures
TMRPNI (RPNI with nerve coaptation to muscle graft motor nerve)	• Provides conduit for reinnervation similar to TMR • Similar donor site morbidity and muscle volume loss to standard RPNI	• Increased technical complexity requiring nerve coaptation (similar to TMR)

preferentially harvested from the amputated specimen, when possible. Recognizing the uncertain relevance of target vascularity, we have increasingly used a strategy whereby pure sensory nerves are provided a denervated, but vascularly intact, nerve interface through burial of the transected proximal nerve into a segment of intact muscle that has been proximally denervated in the course of performing conventional TMR. This "in situ" vascularized RPNI strategy is commonly used for management of sural or posterior femoral cutaneous nerves in conjunction with transtibial or transfemoral TMR, respectively. This hybrid technique is particularly useful in the traumatic or dysvascular setting, where muscle graft revascularization has been questioned. Finally, on several occasions, we have been presented with a residual limb marked by diffuse muscle denervation but symptomatic neuroma pain. Faced with a need to harvest muscle from a separate body area, we have leveraged the segmental innervation of the sartorius muscle[34] to produce muscle grafts that each possess recipient nerves that can be used for direct nerve coaptation with

the donor nerve. We then proceed per our TMR technique as summarized above, but using the small, free nerve-muscle graft. We refer to this technique as TMRPNI, as it uses essentially an RPNI graft with a TMR technique. Although the relative advantage TMRPNI provides compared with conventional RPNI remains unclear as of this writing, this hybrid technique does provide the nerve conduit that conventional RPNI lacks. Furthermore, the added complexity of harvest and coaptation is minimal when a separate muscle harvest site is required.

Neuroma Prevention: Primary Setting

Our overall approach to nerve interface uses in the amputation setting aims to balance the benefits, morbidity, and complexity of these interventions to achieve optimal pain and functional outcomes, while limiting the extent and duration of the operation (Table 2). Given the volume of combat-associated amputees treated at our institution and the role of the Department of Defense in funding neuroma-related research, our center was one

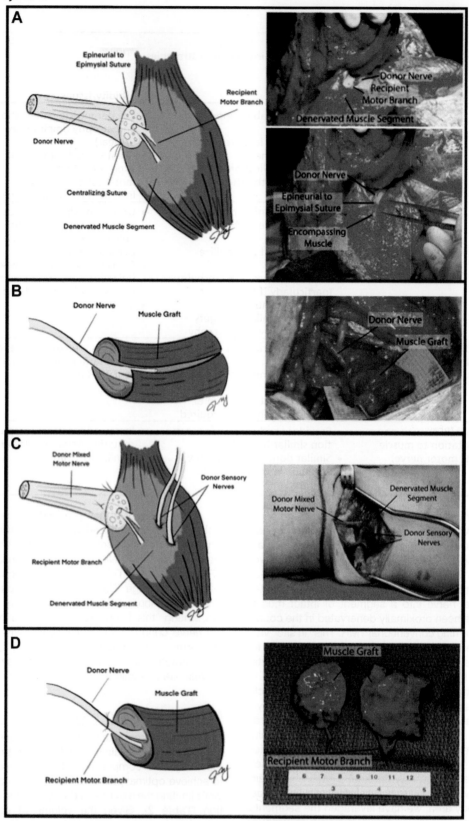

Fig. 2. Illustrated nerve interface strategies with corresponding intraoperative photographs. (*A*) TMR. The donor nerve is coapted to a transected motor branch corresponding to denervated muscle or muscle segment. (*B*) RPNI. The donor nerve is wrapped in a denervated, devascularized muscle graft. (*C*) vRPNI. The donor nerve is buried within vascularized muscle that has been otherwise denervated. (*D*) TMRPNI. The donor nerve is coapted to a transected motor branch corresponding to denervated, devascularized muscle graft.

Table 2
Pearls, pitfalls, and positioning for primary neuroma prevention

Amputation Level	Strategy	Nerves & Targets to Consider in Algorithm	Positioning
Transhumeral	• TMR • RPNI for ulnar nerve if brachialis absent	• Median nerve: either biceps • Ulnar nerve: brachialis • Radial nerve: lateral triceps	• Supine with arm board
Transradial	• TMR	• Median nerve: flexor pronator wad • Ulnar nerve: flexor pronator wad • SBRN: extensor or mobile wad • LABCN: mobile wad	• Supine with arm board
Transfemoral	• TMR with intraneural dissection to isolate sciatic nerve divisions • RPNI for PFCN • Consider for saphenous • Ignore: obturator, LFCN, occasionally saphenous	• Tibial nerve (sciatic): semimembranosus • CPN (sciatic): biceps femoris • PFCN: RPNI, vRPNI to hamstring (denervated by sciatic TMR), or TMR to hamstring motor branch of tibial nerve	• Supine with hip flexed (preferred) • Prone (uncommon)
Transtibial	• TMR • RPNI for sural • Consider RPNI for saphenous	• Tibial nerve: soleus, lateral gastrocnemius, PT • DPN: preserve motor branch to tibialis anterior • SPN: EDL or EHL (motor branch of DPN) • Sural nerves: vRPNI to soleus (denervated by tibial TMR), TMRPNI to tibial motor stump, RPNI, can consider TMR to FHL, gastrocnemius • Saphenous nerve: RPNI	• "Floppy" lateral (preferred) • Prone

Abbreviations: CPN, common peroneal nerve; DPN, deep peroneal nerve; LABCN, lateral antebrachial cutaneous nerve; LFCN, lateral femoral cutaneous nerve; PFCN, posterior femoral cutaneous nerve; SBRN, superficial branch of radial nerve; SPN, superficial peroneal nerve; TMRPNI, targeted muscle regenerative peripheral nerve interface.

of the first to use TMR as a means to treat neuroma-related pain.[6] TMR remains our preferred option for both primary prevention and secondary management of neuroma pain based on our past experience with its use, the size of the vascularized muscle targets, and the strength of the available literature relative to RPNI. RPNI is used in place of TMR when the transected nerve is of poor quality or insufficient length to perform TMR, when no expendable target is available, or when TMR-related denervation atrophy is anticipated to be clinically problematic.

Use of TMR and RPNI in the primary amputation setting is informed by a recent review of patients presenting for secondary neuroma management.[35] We identified a predictable pattern of nerve symptoms based on amputation level. Transfemoral amputees presenting for delayed intervention experienced symptoms almost exclusively from

the sciatic nerve, whereas transtibial amputees most commonly experienced problematic neurologic symptoms emanating from the tibial and peroneal nerves. This predictable pattern of neuroma pain has been used to formulate a targeted approach to neuroma prevention. TMR is applied prophylactically to the most frequently symptomatic nerves, whereas RPNI is used as a conceptually analogous, less morbid, and technically simpler technique for neuroma prevention in less problematic nerves or those less suited to TMR. Although the functional impact of TMR-related residual limb atrophy has yet to be adequately delineated, we have found it to be problematic in a small number of patients, and it is frequently cited as a potential downside of TMR.[36] Regardless, the muscle atrophy that results from TMR is acceptable when weighed against TMR's significant pain benefit. However, we believe the cost-benefit calculation to be different in the prophylactic setting, where TMR performed for all transected nerves would yield more widespread atrophy and the relative pain benefit in a preoperatively asymptomatic patient diminishes. In the lower extremity, TMR is performed for the sciatic, tibial, and peroneal nerves, whereas RPNI is chiefly used for management of the saphenous, sural nerve, and posterior femoral cutaneous nerves.

An important feature of our approach for prophylactic TMR and/or RPNI is the exposure used to access the motor branches. The typical incision and exposure for a lower-extremity amputation does not provide good visualization of the target motor branches, and when they are identifiable, there is a risk of performing a nerve "transfer to nowhere": a motor nerve with most or all of the distal neuromuscular junction and target discarded. We

perform a more proximally based incision for these levels, posterolaterally at the transtibial level, and posteriorly at the transfemoral level. This incision also positions the nerve and the interface away from the terminal aspect of the residuum where it may be compressed by prosthesis wear and weightbearing.

Neuroma Management: Secondary Setting

In the secondary/neuroma management setting, we perform nerve interface procedures for all symptomatic nerves and will additionally address a minimally symptomatic or asymptomatic nerve if it can be accessed through minimal additional exposure and is otherwise known to be a common source of neuroma pain (**Table 3**). We have found that exclusively addressing the most symptomatic

Table 3
Pearls, pitfalls, and positioning for secondary neuroma management

Amputation Level	Strategy	Nerves & Targets to Consider in Algorithm	Positioning
Transhumeral	• TMR for symptomatic nerves • RPNI for ulnar nerve if brachialis absent	• Median nerve: biceps • Ulnar nerve: brachialis • Radial nerve: triceps	• Supine with arm board
Transradial	• TMR for symptomatic nerves	• Median nerve: flexor pronator wad • Ulnar nerve: flexor pronator wad • LABCN: mobile wad • SBRN: extensor or mobile wad	• Supine with arm board
Transfemoral	• TMR for symptomatic nerves • Intraneural dissection to isolate sciatic nerve branches • RPNI for PFCN • RPNI for saphenous if symptomatic • Ignore: obturator, LFCN	• Sciatic nerve (proximal): gluteus maximus • Tibial nerve (sciatic): semimembranosus • CPN (sciatic): biceps femoris • Femoral nerve: quadriceps • PFCN: RPNI, vRPNI to hamstring (denervated by sciatic TMR), or TMR to hamstring motor branch of tibial nerve	• Prone
Transtibial	• TMR for symptomatic nerves • RPNI for sural/ saphenous if symptomatic	• Tibial nerve: soleus, lateral gastrocnemius • Peroneal nerves: preserve DPN to tibialis anterior; CPN/SPN to EDL or EHL (motor branch of DPN) • Sural nerves: vRPNI to soleus (denervated by tibial TMR), TMRPNI to tibial motor stump, RPNI, TMR to FHL, gastrocnemius • Saphenous nerve: RPNI	• Prone or lateral • Lateral preferred (but limits access to saphenous if symptomatic)

nerve can unmask other symptomatic nerves, resulting in an ostensibly successful procedure that nonetheless generates an eventual revision surgery to address other nerves, none more so than when an asymptomatic tibial nerve is left alone in the transtibial amputation setting. As with primary prevention strategies, TMR and RPNI strategies are balanced to limit dissection and operative time. Often, we will consider RPNI for the asymptomatic nerves addressed in this setting.

As previously discussed, TMR is associated with donor muscle atrophy, which may be clinically problematic. For transtibial amputations, where the tibialis anterior is an important component of the terminal limb padding, denervation atrophy may lead to pain with prosthesis wear and poor functional results. To prevent this, we have shifted toward performing intrafascicular dissection to identify and preserve the deep peroneal nerve to tibialis anterior and transferring the superficial peroneal nerve to the distal motor units of the deep peroneal nerve. Results of this strategy appear favorable but have not been objectively measured to this point.

SUMMARY

Although direct myoelectric control is currently limited to upper-extremity prostheses outside of the laboratory, TMR and RPNI are performed in extremity amputees to relieve or prevent neuroma-related and phantom pain and, as a result, potentially improve both patient quality of life and function. In the absence of a comprehensive understanding of the underlying mechanism behind the improved pain outcomes reported with TMR and RPNI, we are limited in our ability to compare the efficacy of the techniques or identify the critical elements beyond the importance of providing a denervated target. Consequently, we have aimed to use the available literature and our institutional experience to formulate a strategy that balances the risks and benefits of each technique and to develop hybrid techniques that deliver the advantages of both where conceptually appropriate.

CLINICS CARE POINTS

- Nerve interface strategies include targeted muscle reinnervation, regenerative peripheral nerve interface, and hybrid techniques, which can be applied to balance surgical goals, complexity, and morbidity to fit the clinical scenario.
- For nerve interfaces procedures to be successful, the nerve requires a distal target and

neurotropic signals. The importance of a conduit is uncertain at this time but can be incorporated into the regenerative peripheral nerve interface technique.

- In the primary setting, a strategy focused on commonly symptomatic nerves results in good long-term pain outcomes while limiting morbidity of unnecessary nerve interface procedures.
- In the delayed setting, nerve interface strategies should target both symptomatic nerves and nerves known to be commonly problematic, as these may be unmasked by addressing the primary cause of pain.

CONFLICT-OF-INTEREST STATEMENT

Each author certifies that he/she has no commercial associations (eg, consultancies, stock ownership, equity interest, patent/licensing arrangements) that might pose a conflict of interest in connection with the submitted article.

All authors are employees of the US Government. This work was prepared as part of their official duties. Title 17 U.S.C. §105 provides that "Copyright protection under this title is not available for any work of the United States Government." Title 17 U.S.C. §101 defined a US Government work as a work prepared by a military service member or employees of the US Government as part of that person's official duties. The opinions or assertions contained herein are the private views of the authors and are not to be construed as reflecting the views, policy, or positions of the Department of Defense, the Uniformed Services University of the Health Sciences, or any other agency of the US Government.

REFERENCES

1. Dumanian GA, Potter BK, Mioton LM, et al. Targeted muscle reinnervation treats neuroma and phantom pain in major limb amputees: a randomized clinical trial. Ann Surg 2019;270(2):238–46.
2. Herr H, Clites T, Srinivasan S, et al. Reinventing extremity amputation in the era of functional limb restoration. Ann Surg 2020;273(2):269–79.
3. Soroush M, Modirian E, Soroush M, et al. Neuroma in bilateral upper limb amputation. Orthopedics 2008; 31(12):1–3.
4. Buchheit T, Ven TV, Hsia H, et al. Pain phenotypes and associated clinical risk factors following traumatic amputation: results from Veterans Integrated Pain Evaluation Research (VIPER): pain phenotypes and associated clinical risk factors. Pain Med 2015;17(1):149–61.

5. Kuiken T, Dumanian G, Lipschutz R, et al. The use of targeted muscle reinnervation for improved myoelectric prosthesis control in a bilateral shoulder disarticulation amputee. Prosthet Orthot Int 2004;28(3):245–53.

6. Daugherty THF, Bueno RA, Neumeister MW. Novel use of targeted muscle reinnervation in the hand for treatment of recurrent symptomatic neuromas following digit amputations. Plast Reconstr Surg Glob Open 2019;7(8):e2376.

7. Souza JM, Cheesborough JE, Ko JH, et al. Targeted muscle reinnervation: a novel approach to postamputation neuroma pain. Clin Orthop Relat Res 2014;472(10):2984–90.

8. Woo SL, Kung TA, Brown DL, et al. Regenerative peripheral nerve interfaces for the treatment of postamputation neuroma pain: a pilot study. Plast Reconstr Surg Glob Open 2016;4(12):e1038.

9. Kubiak C, Kemp S, Cederna P, et al. Prophylactic regenerative peripheral nerve interfaces to prevent postamputation pain. Plast Reconstr Surg 2019;144(3):421e–30e.

10. Valerio IL, Dumanian GA, Jordan SW, et al. Preemptive treatment of phantom and residual limb pain with targeted muscle reinnervation at the time of major limb amputation. J Am Coll Surg 2019;228(3):217–26.

11. Menorca RMG, Fussell TS, Elfar JC. Nerve physiology. Hand Clin 2013;29(3):317–30.

12. Ballantyne JC, Mao J. Opioid therapy for chronic pain. N Engl J Med 2003;349(20):1943–53.

13. Oliveira KMC, Pindur L, Han Z, et al. Time course of traumatic neuroma development. PLoS One 2018; 13(7):e0200548.

14. Gordon T. The physiology of neural injury and regeneration: the role of neurotrophic factors. J Commun Disord 2010;43(4):265–73.

15. Guse DM, Moran SL. Outcomes of the surgical treatment of peripheral neuromas of the hand and forearm: a 25-year comparative outcome study. Ann Plast Surg 2013;71(6):654–8.

16. Eberlin KR, Ducic I. Surgical algorithm for neuroma management: a changing treatment paradigm. Plast Reconstr Surg Glob Open 2018;6(10):e1952.

17. Bergmeister KD, Aman M, Muceli S, et al. Peripheral nerve transfers change target muscle structure and function. Sci Adv 2019;5(1):eaau2956.

18. Omura T, Sano M, Omura K, et al. Different expressions of BDNF, NT3, and NT4 in muscle and nerve after various types of peripheral nerve injuries. J Peripher Nerv Syst 2005;10(3):293–300.

19. Baker J, Constantinescu M, Jones N. Effects of local continuous release of brain derived neurotrophic factor (BDNF) on peripheral nerve regeneration in a rat model. Exp Neurol 2006;199(2):348–53.

20. Dellon AL, Mackinnon SE. Treatment of the painful neuroma by neuroma resection and muscle implantation. Plast Reconstr Surg 1986;77(3):427–36.

21. Kim P, Ko J, O'Shaughnessy K, et al. The effects of targeted muscle reinnervation on neuromas in a rabbit rectus abdominis flap model. J Hand Surg 2012;37(8):1609–16.

22. Amir R, Devor M. Ongoing activity in neuroma afferents bearing retrograde sprouts. Brain Res 1993; 630(1–2):283–8.

23. Urbanchek MG, Kung TA, Frost CM, et al. Development of a regenerative peripheral nerve interface for control of a neuroprosthetic limb. Biomed Res Int 2016;2016:1–8.

24. Sakai Y, Ochi M, Uchio Y, et al. Prevention and treatment of amputation neuroma by an atelocollagen tube in rat sciatic nerves. J Biomed Mater Res B Appl Biomater 2005;73B(2):355–60.

25. Valerio I, Schulz SA, West J, et al. Targeted muscle reinnervation combined with a vascularized pedicled regenerative peripheral nerve interface. Plast Reconstr Surg Glob Open 2020;8(3):e2689.

26. Szczesny G, Veihelmann A, Nolte D, et al. Changes in the local blood and lymph microcirculation in response to direct mechanical trauma applied to leg: in vivo study in an animal model. J Trauma Acute Care 2001;51(3):508–17.

27. Hu Y, Sando IC, Cederna PS, et al. Impact of muscle graft volume on signaling capacity in the regenerative peripheral nerve interface for neuroprosthetic control. Plast Reconstr Surg 2015;136(4 Suppl):38–9.

28. Srinivasan S, Diaz M, Carty M, et al. Towards functional restoration for persons with limb amputation: a dual-stage implementation of regenerative agonist-antagonist myoneural interfaces. Sci Rep 2019;9(1):1981.

29. Levinson S, Luo S, Henry M. The role of sodium channels in chronic pain. Muscle Nerve 2012; 46(2):155–65.

30. Du X, Gamper N. Potassium channels in peripheral pain pathways: expression, function and therapeutic potential. Curr Neuropharmacol 2013;11(6):621–40.

31. Moore A, Macewan M, Santosa K, et al. Acellular nerve allografts in peripheral nerve regeneration: a comparative study. Muscle Nerve 2011;44(2):221–34.

32. Bowen J, Wee C, Kalik J, et al. Targeted muscle reinnervation to improve pain, prosthetic tolerance, and bioprosthetic outcomes in the amputee. Adv Wound Care 2017;6(8):261–7.

33. Kubiak C, Kemp S, Cederna P. Regenerative peripheral nerve interface for management of postamputation neuroma. JAMA Surg 2018;153(7):681.

34. Yang D, Morris SF, Sigurdson L. The sartorius muscle: anatomic considerations for reconstructive surgeons. Surg Radiol Anat 1998;20(5):307–10.

35. Hoyt B, Potter BK, Souza JM. Practice patterns and pain outcomes for targeted muscle reinnervation: an informed approach to targeted muscle reinnervation use in the acute amputation setting. J Bone Joint Surg Am 2021;103(8):681–7.

36. Lineaweaver W, Zhang F. Clarifying the role of targeted muscle reinnervation in amputation management. J Am Coll Surg 2019;229(6):635.

Dermatosensory Peripheral Nerve Interfaces: Prevention of Pain Recurrence Following Sensory Neurectomy

Sarah E. Hart, MD, David L. Brown, MD*

KEYWORDS

- DSPNI • Neuroma • Neuropathic pain • Dermatosensory • Peripheral nerve interface
- Chronic pain

KEY POINTS

- When chronic pain (ie, pain lasting >3 months) results after injury or operation, a neuropathic origin should be considered.
- Neuropathic pain can be highly suspected through history (eg, pain character, timing of onset, and location) and physical examination (eg, changes in sensation, pinpoint tenderness, Tinel sign).
- Confirmation of involved nerves and associated neuromas can be achieved with blind or ultrasonography-guided nerve blocks.
- New procedures that provide physiologic targets for regenerating axons following nerve transection show promise in improving pain outcomes.
- Dermatosensory peripheral nerve interfaces may provide the optimal environment to prevent recurrence of chronic pain following neurectomy.

BACKGROUND

Chronic pain is a monumental health concern, affecting more people than heart disease and cancer combined.[1] Advances in the diagnosis of neuropathic pain and techniques for localizing nerve injury have led to improvements in the ability to treat many chronic pain conditions. Neurectomy is currently the mainstay of surgical treatment of neuropathic pain. A neuroma occurs following peripheral nerve transection, when nerve regeneration does not result in the reinnervation of a distal target, and instead results in disorganized axonal sprouting. Neuromas can show ectopic neural activity and hypersensitivity to both mechanical and chemical stimulation.[2] Therefore, many neuromas become symptomatic and contribute to clinically significant, chronic neuropathic pain.

Conventional treatment of symptomatic neuromas includes both nonsurgical and surgical modalities. Nonsurgical treatments include desensitization therapy, local anesthetic injections, transcutaneous electrical nerve stimulation, pain catheters, and pharmacologic management.[3–5] Surgical management of neuropathic symptoms has been shown to have higher efficacy,[6] and many surgical approaches have been proposed. One of the earliest techniques involves transposing a painful neuroma into a nearby muscle belly in an attempt to move it to a protected location, less likely to be irritated by external mechanical stimuli.[7,8] Another early technique

Section of Plastic Surgery, Department of Surgery, University of Michigan Medical School, 1500 E Medical Center Drive, 2130 Taubman Center, Ann Arbor, MI 48109, USA
* Corresponding author.
E-mail address: davbrown@med.umich.edu

Hand Clin 37 (2021) 383–389
https://doi.org/10.1016/j.hcl.2021.05.005
0749-0712/21/© 2021 Elsevier Inc. All rights reserved.

involves neuroma excision with traction neurec-tomy.[9] This technique does not prevent neuroma recurrence, but it does encourage potential recurrence at a more protected proximal location less prone to stimulation. Subsequent techniques were designed with the goal of preventing distal axonal regeneration. More than 100 techniques have been reported[8,10] and include cauterization or freezing of the proximal nerve end,[11,12] suturing epineurium over the distal stump,[12] application of ricin to result in retrograde axonal so-called sui-cide transport,[13–15] and the widely popularized transposition of the nerve end into muscle, vein, or bone.[6,16–18] However, these techniques often yield incomplete pain relief or recurrence of symptomatic neuroma pain[9,19] with high reoperation rates.[6] A recent meta-analysis of 54 studies evaluating these traditional surgical interventions reported that 20% to 30% of symptomatic neuromas were refractory to surgical treatment regardless of the surgery performed.[6] The lack of success in reliably treating symptomatic neuroma pain using current methods that attempt to thwart axonal regeneration has led to a paradigm shift toward treatment modalities that capitalize on physiologic processes to prevent neuroma formation.

REINNERVATION OF DENERVATED TARGETS TO PREVENT NEUROMA FORMATION

Two novel surgical techniques have been developed that leverage nerve regeneration and reinnervation in order to address symptomatic neuromas: targeted muscle reinnervation (TMR) and regenerative peripheral nerve interface (RPNI).[20,21] In contrast with the previously described techniques that focus on attempting to physically curtail or misdirect axonal growth, these new methods purposefully facilitate reinnervation of specific distal targets. The downstream target for TMR is a nearby motor nerve branch leading to a segment of denervated muscle fibers within a local muscle.[22] In comparison, the physiologic end point for RPNI is a denervated free muscle graft.[23] By offering regenerating axons distal targets for reinnervation, both of these techniques allow natural physiologic processes to occur. Therefore, by facilitating reinnervation of denervated targets, these strategies reduce the number of aimless axons at the end of a transected nerve that are available to reform a symptomatic neuroma.

It is well known that peripheral nerves show preferential targeted reinnervation: sensory axons have an innate predilection for innervation of sensory end organs and motor axons for neuromuscular junctions. Numerous studies have shown that regenerating motor axons create functional neuromuscular junctions within denervated muscle,[24–28] whereas regenerating sensory axons innervate sensory targets such as muscle spindles and Golgi tendon organs.[29–34] Given this preferential reinnervation, transected nerves containing afferent sensory axons may best be treated by providing dermal sensory end organs, as is the case when primary nerve repair is possible.

The dermatosensory peripheral nerve interface (DSPNI) uses a deepithelialized dermal graft as the physiologic end point for sensory nerve regeneration. In this technique, the epineurium of the freshly divided nerve end is secured to an autologous dermal graft using fine monofilament suture. The graft is then wrapped or folded around the nerve end, completely enveloping it, and is secured in this position with additional sutures (**Fig. 1**). The DSPNI method is a variation of the RPNI, except that a free dermal graft is used instead of a free muscle graft. Some early evidence suggests that RPNIs may be successful in reducing neuropathic pain caused by neuromas involving sensory nerves,[35] presumably because of sensory axon reinnervation of sensory targets within the muscle graft.[36] Therefore, a dermal graft would be an even more appropriate denervated target for regenerating axons within a transected sensory nerve. Preliminary research has shown successful reinnervation of dermal grafts by showing the elicitation of afferent compound

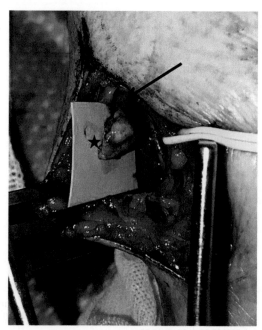

Fig. 1. Example of a DSPNI (*star*) on the proximal nerve end (*arrow*), after resection of a cutaneous nerve.

sensory nerve action potentials following electrical stimulation of the grafts.[37–40] In addition, histomorphometric analysis of the dermal sensory interfaces showed no evidence of neuroma formation as well as minimal inflammation and complete viability of the dermis through revascularization.[37,40] Furthermore, immunohistochemistry has shown successful reinnervation of sensory end organs within dermal grafts.[38]

The DSPNI technique can be used in patients presenting with chronic pain of neuropathic origin whose symptoms and corresponding physical examination can be localized to a specific sensory nerve. Two common, ideal patient populations include chronic neuropathic pain following lower extremity injury and/or orthopedic surgery, as well as mastectomy and/or breast reconstruction. The following 2 cases highlight our preferred perioperative work-up and intraoperative treatment of these patients.

CASE STUDY 1: SUPERFICIAL PERONEAL AND SAPHENOUS NEURECTOMIES WITH DERMATOSENSORY PERIPHERAL NERVE INTERFACES FOR LOWER EXTREMITY PAIN

A 57-year-old woman presented with 17 months of chronic left foot and ankle pain following an inversion injury managed nonoperatively by a foot and ankle specialist. She was worked up and cleared of any structural issues. She reported subjective numbness of the dorsum of her foot as well as intermittent shooting pain down the medial and lateral aspects of the ankle and foot that radiated toward the second and third toes. The pain interfered with her normal activities and work. Her visual analog score (VAS) pain rating at her initial clinic visit was 6 out of 10, with her worst pain in the last 2 weeks rated as 9 out of 10.

On physical examination, there was decreased sensation (6 out of 10) over the dorsal foot in the distribution of the superficial peroneal nerve (SPN), 7 out of 10 in between the great and second toes in the distribution of the deep peroneal nerve, and normal sensation in the sural, saphenous, and tibial nerve distributions, compared with the contralateral limb. There was a positive Tinel sign along the SPN, approximately 4 cm proximal to the lateral malleolus, and this painful signal intensified as percussion moved distally along the course of the nerve onto the foot. The remaining examination was normal with 2+ pedal pulses, full active range of motion of the ankle, and full strength with ankle dorsiflexion, plantarflexion, eversion, and inversion.

Given concern for a traction injury to the SPN from her previous ankle inversion, a local anesthetic block was performed blindly in the clinic using 0.5% bupivacaine mixed with 1% lidocaine with epinephrine 1:100,000 to the left SPN, above the location of the Tinel sign. The block resulted in complete numbness of the dorsum of the foot, confirming success of the block. Full resolution of her pain was reported 10 minutes later. Given the success of this targeted diagnostic local anesthetic block, neurectomy of the SPN with DSPNI was offered to the patient.

On the day of surgery, the location of the proximal most extent of the Tinel sign over the left SPN was marked and confirmed with the patient. General anesthesia was induced, and she was positioned supine with her left extremity flexed at the knee. A 5-cm elliptical excision was made, centered 10 cm above the lateral malleolus, overlying the lateral compartment (marked one-quarter of the way between the fibula and the lateral edge of the tibia). The ellipse of skin was deepithelialized and a dermal graft was separated from the underlying fat and preserved. Dissection was carried down to the muscle fascia and the area of perforation of the lateral compartment fascia by the SPN was identified. The SPN was visualized to be diminutive, appearing approximately 30% of its expected diameter. Therefore, the anterior compartment was explored for a second branch of the SPN (present in approximately 25% of cases[41]), which was identified. Both branches of the proximal SPN were dissected free from the surrounding soft tissue and muscle. Infiltration of 0.5% bupivacaine was performed proximal to the planned level of transection several minutes before neurectomy as a form of preemptive analgesia. Anesthetizing the nerve before transection blocks the activation of peripheral nervous system pain pathways, limiting the trauma experienced by the central nervous system. Preemptive analgesia prevents the establishment of altered processing of future sensory inputs that could amplify postoperative pain.[42] Sharp transection and removal of 2 to 3 cm of each nerve segment was performed, and the proximal nerve ends were wrapped with 1 × 2-cm dermal grafts as described previously (Fig. 2). A 2-cm to 3-cm segment of nerve was excised to impede the propensity for the proximal nerve end to attempt to regrow to the distal end. The DSPNIs were then pushed proximally along the course of the respective nerves, creating laxity to prevent distal scar tethering, a potential cause of recurrent stimulation. Following wound closure, the leg was wrapped with a compressive wrap. Nerve protocol medications consisting of a single 300-mg dose of gabapentin preoperatively, low-dose ketamine intraoperatively, and a postoperative regimen of

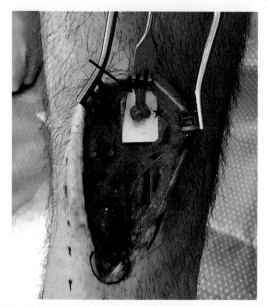

Fig. 2. Neurectomy of a neuromatous SPN (*arrow*) with DSPNI of the proximal end (*star*).

acetaminophen 500 mg twice a day for 2 weeks, gabapentin 300 mg twice a day and vitamin C 500 mg twice a day for 3 months, and oxycodone 5 mg (10 pills total) for breakthrough pain was used.[43] Postoperative mobility was not restricted.

At 1 week following surgery, the patient reported significant improvement in her pain symptoms (now 2 out of 10). At her 3-month follow-up, she described new burning, 8 out of 10 pain on the dorsomedial aspect of her left ankle and foot. Her initial pain in the SPN distribution continued to be significantly improved. On examination, she had numbness of the dorsal foot consistent with SPN neurectomy, as well as a positive Tinel sign over the left saphenous nerve in the medial lower leg.

We hypothesize that the saphenous nerve likely sustained a traction injury at the time of her ankle inversion, resulting in a neuroma in continuity and resultant pain. Symptoms from the SPN injury were potentially more significant and distracted from the separate localization of pain from the saphenous nerve. With the SPN neuropathic pain now treated, the saphenous nerve disorder was unmasked. A block of the saphenous nerve resolved her new pain and saphenous neurectomy with DSPNI was planned.

An entirely similar operation to the original was performed on the saphenous nerve (with neurectomy and DSPNI above the level of tenderness and Tinel sign) in the distal third of the lower leg. At 1 week postoperatively, she reported much improved pain in the saphenous nerve distribution,

ranked 3 out of 10 (from 8 out of 10), and her physical examination revealed no Tinel sign. After 6 weeks, she had returned to her normal activities without complications.

CASE STUDY 2: INTERCOSTAL NEURECTOMY AND DERMATOSENSORY PERIPHERAL NERVE INTERFACE FOR CHRONIC BREAST PAIN

A 41-year-old woman complained of chronic left lateral breast pain following bilateral mastectomies and immediate breast reconstruction with a right latissimus flap and tissue expanders ultimately exchanged for bilateral silicone implants. She could pinpoint the epicenter of the pain to a location on the left lateral breast. The pain limited her daily activities, including laundry and housework. Her VAS pain score was a 10. Pertinent daily medications included naproxen, ibuprofen, tramadol, and venlafaxine.

On physical examination, she showed significant tenderness to palpation and Tinel signs at each of the rib interspaces in the midaxillary line, from T2 through T5. A local anesthetic block was performed blindly in the office using 0.5% bupivacaine mixed with 1% lidocaine with epinephrine 1:100,000. At each level from T2 to T5, 2 mL of the local anesthetic mixture was injected into the deep subcutaneous space/muscle fascia level along the midaxillary line at the presumed location of the lateral intercostal nerve branches. She described subjective numbness to light touch of the lateral breast, confirming a successful nerve block. After the diagnostic local anesthetic block, her VAS score decreased to 0 and manual palpation of the involved intercostal spaces and of the lateral breast elicited no tenderness. The combination of her history, physical examination, and nerve block result confirmed the diagnosis of neuropathic pain caused by injury to the lateral cutaneous branches of intercostal nerves T2 through T5, located distal to the penetration of the nerves through the muscular fascia. Injury could be presumed to be caused by end neuromas or neuromas-in-continuity of these nerve branches from direct cutting or thermal injury, retraction stretch, and/or scar entrapment. Neurectomy of lateral sensory intercostal nerves at T2, T3, T4, and T5 with DSPNI creation was recommended.

On the day of surgery, the involved lateral cutaneous intercostal nerves were again identified by physical examination, confirmed with the patient, and marked. General anesthesia was used, and she was placed in a right lateral decubitus position. A vertical elliptical incision was made in the midaxillary line, and a dermal graft was harvested as in the previous case. Dissection down to the

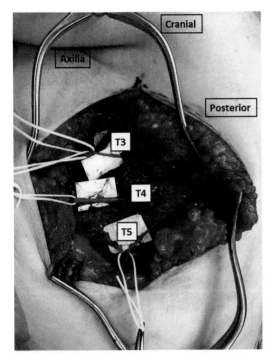

Fig. 3. Example of dissection of lateral intercostal sensory nerves at T3, T4, and T5, in the midaxillary line. Note anterior and posterior branches, particularly well highlighted at T5.

muscle fascia using Metzenbaum scissors was performed to identify one of the anterior or posterior intercostal branches, which was then traced proximally to the main lateral division as it penetrated up through the muscle fascia. Additional lateral divisions were located in the adjacent rib interspaces, directly in a vertical line from the first identified nerve (**Fig. 3**). Infiltration of 0.5% bupivacaine was performed into each nerve at the level of the fascia several minutes before neurectomy for preemptive analgesia. Resection of 2 to 3 cm of nerve was performed at the level of the fascia, and the proximal nerve ends were each wrapped with a DSPNI. Wrapped nerve ends were buried deep along the course of the proximal nerve, to prevent scar tethering. As detailed earlier, a medication nerve protocol was used.

Postoperatively, the patient had significant improvement in her pain symptoms. At 3 months, she reported her pain as 1 out of 10. She returned to her normal activities without complications.

SUMMARY

The DSPNI is a variation of the RPNI and it provides an optimal method to treat and prevent neuroma pain following sensory nerve transection by permitting sensory nerve regeneration and reinnervation of denervated dermal grafts. The effective treatment of neuropathic pain has the potential to lead to transformative reductions in the number of patients living with chronic pain. The surgical technique of DSPNI is a straightforward outpatient operation with a low complication profile and low patient morbidity. All patients presenting with chronic neuropathic pain from suspected nerve injury should be considered for DSPNI surgery.

CLINICS CARE POINTS

- Patients complaining of burning, stabbing, or shocklike pain following injury or an operation should be evaluated for a neuropathic cause.
- Localized nerve blocks can confirm which nerve is involved, and an improvement in pain complaints following the block is an indication for operative intervention.
- Procedures that provide physiologic targets for regenerating axons may combat neuropathic pain. Muscle grafts are ideal for motor or mixed nerves, whereas dermal grafts are ideal for sensory nerves. The predilection of these nerve types for their respective targets has been shown.
- DSPNI is a new technique that provides the optimal environment to prevent chronic neuropathic pain following neurectomy.

DISCLOSURE

The authors have nothing to disclose.

REFERENCES

1. Dahlhamer J, Lucas J, Zelaya C, et al. Prevalence of chronic pain and high-impact chronic pain among adults - United States, 2016. MMWR Morb Mortal Wkly Rep 2018;67(36):1001–6.
2. Hsu E, Cohen SP. Postamputation pain: epidemiology, mechanisms, and treatment. J Pain Res 2013;6:121–36.
3. van der Avoort DJ, Hovius SE, Selles RW, et al. The incidence of symptomatic neuroma in amputation and neurorrhaphy patients. J Plast Reconstr Aesthet Surg 2013;66(10):1330–4.

4. Stokvis A, van der Avoort DJ, van Neck JW, et al. Surgical management of neuroma pain: a prospective follow-up study. Pain 2010;151(3):862–9.

5. Wolvetang NHA, Lans J, Verhiel SHWL, et al. Surgery for symptomatic neuroma: anatomic distribution and predictors of secondary surgery. Plast Reconstr Surg 2019;143(6):1762–71.

6. Poppler LH, Parikh RP, Bichanich MJ, et al. Surgical interventions for the treatment of painful neuroma: a comparative meta-analysis. Pain 2018;159(2): 214–23.

7. Herndon JH, Eaton RG, Littler JW. Management of painful neuromas in the hand. J Bone Joint Surg Am 1976;58(3):369–73.

8. Dellon AL, Aszmann OC. In musculus, veritas? Nerve "in muscle" versus targeted muscle reinnervation versus regenerative peripheral nerve interface: historical review. Microsurgery 2020;40(4): 516–22.

9. Ducic I, Mesbahi AN, Attinger CE, et al. The role of peripheral nerve surgery in the treatment of chronic pain associated with amputation stumps. Plast Reconstr Surg 2008;121(3):908–14 [discussion 915-7].

10. Elliot D. Surgical management of painful peripheral nerves. Clin Plast Surg 2014;41(3):589–613.

11. Swanson AB, Boeve NR, Lumsden RM. The prevention and treatment of amputation neuromata by silicone capping. J Hand Surg Am 1977;2(1):70–8.

12. Tupper JW, Booth DM. Treatment of painful neuromas of sensory nerves in the hand: a comparison of traditional and newer methods. J Hand Surg Am 1976;1(2):144–51.

13. Brandner MD, Buncke HJ, Campagna-Pinto D. Experimental treatment of neuromas in the rat by retrograde axoplasmic transport of ricin with selective destruction of ganglion cells. J Hand Surg Am 1989;14(4):710–4.

14. Nennesmo I, Kristensson K. Effects of retrograde axonal transport of Ricinus communis agglutinin I on neuroma formation. Acta Neuropathol 1986; 70(3–4):279–83.

15. Shapiro S, Voelker J. Reduction of experimental neuroma formation with ricin. J Surg Res 1991;51(5): 405–8.

16. Moszkowicz L. Zur Behandlung der schmerzhaften neurome. Zmtralbl Clair 1918;45:547.

17. Dellon AL, Mackinnon SE, Pestronk A. Implantation of sensory nerve into muscle: preliminary clinical and experimental observations on neuroma formation. Ann Plast Surg 1984;12(1):30–40.

18. Mackinnon SE, Dellon AL, Hudson AR, et al. Alteration of neuroma formation by manipulation of its microenvironment. Plast Reconstr Surg 1985;76(3):345–53.

19. Barberá J, Albert-Pampló R. Centrocentral anastomosis of the proximal nerve stump in the treatment of painful amputation neuromas of major nerves. J Neurosurg 1993;79(3):331–4.

20. Dumanian GA, Potter BK, Mioton LM, et al. Targeted muscle reinnervation treats neuroma and phantom pain in major limb amputees: a randomized clinical trial. Ann Surg 2019;270(2):238–46.

21. Woo SL, Kung TA, Brown DL, et al. Regenerative peripheral nerve interfaces for the treatment of postamputation neuroma pain: a pilot study. Plast Reconstr Surg Glob Open 2016;4(12):e1038.

22. Kuiken TA, Barlow AK, Hargrove L, et al. Targeted muscle reinnervation for the upper and lower extremity. Tech Orthop 2017;32(2):109–16.

23. Urbanchek MG, Kung TA, Frost CM, et al. Development of a regenerative peripheral nerve interface for control of a neuroprosthetic limb. Biomed Res Int 2016;2016:5726730.

24. Bader D. Reinnervation of motor endplate-containing and motor endplate-less muscle grafts. Dev Biol 1980;77(2):315–27.

25. Hakelius L, Nyström B, Stålberg E. Histochemical and neurophysiological studies of autotransplanted cat muscle. Scand J Plast Reconstr Surg 1975; 9(1):15–24.

26. Killer H, Müntener M. Time course of the regeneration of the endplate zone after autologous muscle transplantation. Experientia 1986;42(3):301–2.

27. Dhawan V, Lytle IF, Dow DE, et al. Neurotization improves contractile forces of tissue-engineered skeletal muscle. Tissue Eng 2007;13(11):2813–21.

28. Borschel GH, Dow DE, Dennis RG, et al. Tissue-engineered axially vascularized contractile skeletal muscle. Plast Reconstr Surg 2006;117(7):2235–42.

29. Dellon AL. Muscle sense, or nonsense? Ann Plast Surg 1991;26(5):444–8.

30. Dellon AL, Witebsky FG, Terrill RE. The denervated Meissner corpuscle. A sequential histological study after nerve division in the Rhesus monkey. Plast Reconstr Surg 1975;56(2):182–93.

31. Dellon AL. Reinnervation of denervated Meissner corpuscles: a sequential histologic study in the monkey following fasicular nerve repair. J Hand Surg Am 1976;1(2):98–109.

32. Kuiken TA, Marasco PD, Lock BA, et al. Redirection of cutaneous sensation from the hand to the chest skin of human amputees with targeted reinnervation. Proc Natl Acad Sci U S A 2007;104(50):20061–6.

33. Banks RW, Barker D. Specificities of afferents reinnervating cat muscle spindles after nerve section. J Physiol 1989;408:345–72.

34. Banks RW. The innervation of the muscle spindle: a personal history. J Anat 2015;227(2):115–35.

35. Hooper R, Cederna P, Brown D, et al. Regenerative peripheral nerve interface for the management of symptomatic hand and digital neuromas. Plast Reconstr Surg Glob Open 2020;8(6):e2792.

36. Bain JR, Veltri KL, Chamberlain D, et al. Improved functional recovery of denervated skeletal muscle

after temporary sensory nerve innervation. Neuroscience 2001;103(2):503–10.

37. Sando I, Gerling G, Ursu D, et al. Dermal-based peripheral nerve interface for transduction of sensory feedback. Plast Reconstr Surg 2015;19–20.

38. Svientek SR, Ursu DC, Cederna PS, et al. Fabrication of the Composite Regenerative Peripheral Nerve Interface (C-RPNI) in the adult rat. J Vis Exp 2020;(156).

39. Kubiak C, Ursu D, Moon J, et al. Viability and signal transduction with the composite regenerative peripheral nerve interface (C-RPNI). Plast Reconstr Surg Glob Open 2019;26–7.

40. Larson JV, Urbanchek MG, Moon JD, et al. Abstract 17: prototype sensory regenerative peripheral nerve interface for artificial limb somatosensory feedback. Plast Reconstr Surg 2014;133(3 Suppl):26–7.

41. Barrett SL, Dellon AL, Rosson GD, et al. Superficial peroneal nerve (superficial fibularis nerve): the clinical implications of anatomic variability. J Foot Ankle Surg 2006;45(3):174–6.

42. Kissin I. Preemptive analgesia. Anesthesiology 2000;93(4):1138–43.

43. Carroll I, Hah J, Mackey S, et al. Perioperative interventions to reduce chronic postsurgical pain. J Reconstr Microsurg 2013;29(4):213–22.

Brain-Machine Interfaces
Lessons for Prosthetic Hand Control

Alex K. Vaskov, PhD[a], Cynthia A. Chestek, PhD[a,b,c,d,*]

KEYWORDS

- Brain-machine interfaces • Fine motor control • Regression algorithms • Pattern recognition
- Calibration methods

KEY POINTS

- Brain-machine interfaces (BMI) directly access the nervous system to control arm and hand prostheses.
- BMI control algorithms are highly transferrable to peripheral recording techniques for myoelectric prostheses.
- Researchers investigating both brain-machine interfaces and myoelectric control face similar challenges controlling multiple degrees of freedom and acquiring clean calibration data from patients with injuries or disabilities.
- Solutions to these issues will likely be transferable between the 2 technologies.

INTRODUCTION

The loss of an upper extremity is a devastating injury that severely affects a person's ability to interact with the world around them. Hands remain our primary mechanisms for tool use and are important components of social interaction. Advances in robotics have yielded electronic prostheses that can mimic anywhere from 5 to 30degrees of freedom (DOF) of the human hand and provide adequate gripping force for functional tasks.[1–3] The clinical standard is to control these devices with surface electromyography (EMG), allowing users to use muscle activity for control. Dual-site control schemes are cumbersome and unintuitive, requiring a substituted pair of easily accessible agonist-antagonist muscle groups to trigger switches between hand and wrist movements and modulate single DOF. For some users, state of the art pattern recognition systems have eliminated the need for triggers or movement substitutions, and targeted muscle reinnervation

surgery expanded these benefits to users with more proximal amputations.[4,5] However, simultaneous control of multiple DOF has proved difficult.[6] Intuitive grasp selection has been demonstrated in controlled studies[5,7,8] and has only recently become available in commercial devices.

One of the main challenges of existing systems is the ability to extract specific motor commands from surface EMG, which represents a spatiotemporal summation of motor unit activity.[9] Classifiers, the algorithmic engine of pattern recognition systems, are adept at distinguishing movements from such summaries and can even remain accurate in systems with fewer input channels.[7,8,10] However, scaling to multi-DOF control requires distinguishing a rapidly increasing number of movement combinations. Hierarchical schemes have been proposed to alleviate this issue,[11] but the lack of independent control signals remains problematic.[6] Intuitive grasp and fine motor control is of high interest to prostheses users[12]

This work was supported by the National Institute of Health, award R01NS105132.
[a] Robotics Institute, University of Michigan, 2505 Hayward St, Ann Arbor, MI 48109, USA; [b] Department of Biomedical Engineering, University of Michigan, 2200 Bonisteel Blvd, Ann Arbor, MI 48109, USA; [c] Department of Electrical Engineering and Computer Science, University of Michigan, 1301 Beal Ave, Ann Arbor, MI 48109, USA; [d] Neuroscience Graduate Program, University of Michigan, 204 Washtenaw Ave, Ann Arbor, MI 48109, USA
* Corresponding author.
E-mail address: cchestek@umich.edu

Hand Clin 37 (2021) 391–399
https://doi.org/10.1016/j.hcl.2021.04.003

but is difficult because many muscles responsible for thumb and finger movements are either lost due to the level of amputation or obscured by more superficial muscles. Peripheral nerve interfacing and surgically invasive recording techniques are being proposed to resolve these issues.[13–16] Extracting precise movement commands from electrophysiological activity is paramount to many rehabilitation and neuroprosthetic applications. In some of these cases, researchers are developing implantable devices and algorithms to solve problems that are fundamentally similar to the challenges experienced with traditional myoelectric prosthetic devices. Brain-machine interfaces (BMI) are being explored for movement assistance and control of robotic devices or computers for patient populations including persons suffering severe stroke, spinal-cord injuries (SCI), or amyotrophic lateral sclerosis. Here the authors discuss progress in BMI for neuroprosthetic control and how they could inform development of better implantable EMG control strategies for myoelectric hands.

DISCUSSION
Signal Acquisition

For patients suffering neurodegenerative diseases or injuries, for example, late-stage ALS or high-level SCI, severe damage renders the peripheral nervous system either an impossible or a poor source of information to extract motor commands for prosthetic control. For these applications, researchers are looking to the brain as an information source. The brain is the origin of intended movement commands for arm and hand control, and its somatotopy is reliably consistent between individuals to facilitate targeting these functions. Electroencephalography (EEG) is a noninvasive technique that records electrical brain activity from the surface of the scalp. Although useful for monitoring or diagnostic applications, EEG has not been widely adopted for neuroprosthetic control. The activity of a single neuron is too small to be recorded remotely through the skull, so EEG recorded reflects a summation of the synchronous activity of thousands or millions of pyramidal neurons.[17] The low conductivity of bone and the exponential decrease in voltage gradients as the recording electrode becomes more distant further reduces the signal specificity and lowers the signal to noise ratios (SNR), making signal interpretation difficult.[18] These properties make EEG ill-suited for prosthetic control applications, which require algorithms to confidently estimate, or "decode", movement intentions in real time. Over the past 2 decades, BMI researchers have capitalized on the availability and development of surgically invasive techniques for neuroprosthetic control to eliminate the need to record signals through the bone and improve SNR.

Recent surveys have shown that fast, accurate, and natural control of external prostheses or restoration of natural arm and hand control are priorities for patients with SCI considering surgically invasive procedures.[19,20] For motor control applications, intracortical electrodes have yielded the best performance in both nonhuman primate (NHP) and clinical studies.[21–23] The Utah Electrode Array (Blackrock Microsystems, Salt Lake City, Utah, USA) is clinically available in multiple configurations with 96 to 128 independent electrode shanks that penetrate 1.0 to 1.5 mm into the brain. When implanted into the motor cortex, penetrating shanks capture local field, single neuron, or multi-unit activity reflective of intended movement kinematics and dynamics.[24,25] Access to source signals provides engineers with the opportunity to develop systems that predict and actuate prosthetic devices without exceeding the time delay of natural movement. Neural firing rates can be counted by manual spike sorting to identify individual wave forms,[26] threshold crossings that aggregate units per channel,[27,28] or power in frequency bands that reflects motor neuron firing.[29–31] Signal processing techniques that capture individual neuron activity have yielded the best performance. Low-frequency (<300 Hz), local field potentials may be used to augment firing rates as a stable input but have not proved sufficient as a standalone feature.[32–34] Biological responses to the penetrating electrodes can lead to tissue scarring and cell death, which ultimately reduce signal quality and the longevity of the BMI.[35–37] Novel electrode designs, to minimize scarring and increase biocompatibility, are an active area of research to address this challenge.[38–40] Flexible electrode grids record electrocorticography (ECoG) from the surface of the brain and may alleviate some of the biological risks of penetrating electrodes, although the precision and speed of motor control has been lacking to date.[41] For intracortical and ECoG applications, multiple groups are developing implantable electronics to bring systems closer to clinical reality.[42–45]

For persons with amputations, activity of the peripheral motor system can be monitored via surface EMG and used to command prostheses. Commercially available systems predict movements based on compound muscle activation patterns. Depending on patient anatomy and prostheses capabilities, this approach may be sufficient. However, simultaneous control of wrist joints or dexterous hand functions has proved difficult.[6] Access to movement-specific commands from the neuromuscular system can improve device control. Muscle tissue has proved to be a durable interface for implanted electrodes to record stable EMG for months and years,[14,16,46] and routine surgical techniques have used either transplanted or denervated muscle to provide a stable interface with the nervous system.[4,16,47] Intramuscular EMG is often preprocessed for input into control algorithms by band-pass filtering, rectification, and integration. Bandwidths and processing windows vary across studies but are similar to parameters used to isolate nearby muscle activity in surface EMG.[13,14,16] In a bipolar configuration, the mean absolute value of each filtered channel reflects a highly localized summation of motor unit activity specific to the implanted muscle. Like intracortical electrode grids, intramuscular EMG records motor impulses with a high spatial and temporal resolution. Therefore, it is not surprising that a similar algorithmic framework can be applied to control prostheses from downstream motor units in extremity muscles. This review focuses on intracortical approaches that have enabled dexterous control of natural limbs[48,49] or robotic prostheses.[22,50]

Regression Algorithms

Many patients have positive attitudes regarding invasive BMIs if they provide high levels of performance.[19,20] Most controllers accomplish this with linear regression algorithms that adhere to similar framework. Typically, regressors model the intended position or velocity of DOF as continuous variables that explain neural activity.[21,22,51] The regression algorithm, or "decoder", accepts firing rates as an input and usually outputs velocities in each DOF to control the virtual or physical prostheses. Velocity output is typically used regardless of whether or not neural activity is assumed to be tuned to position[21,52] and is suspected to produce a simple physical system for real-time control in the presence of noisy inputs.[53,54] Researchers have also noticed that executing algorithms on shorter time intervals (<100 ms) improves online performance, which may be contradictory to offline simulations,[55] and this is thought to be due to improvements in both the rate of visual feedback and control rate that improve error correction and movement planning.[23] To date, many BMIs use linear regressions to decode arm reaches, which are then mapped to provide 2 DOF cursor control in a virtual environment. However, clinical trials have demonstrated that the following framework can also be applied to control higher DOF robotic limbs[22,50] or functional electrical stimulation

(FES) systems.[48,49] More recently, both NHP and clinical studies have demonstrated that a linear framework can be extended to precisely control individual finger or grasp dimensions.[31,52,56]

Over the last decade, clinical BMI have most commonly used 2 linear algorithms: optimal linear estimation (OLE) with ridge regression and the Kalman filter (KF).[22,50] In the early 2000s, the first linear regressors in NHP used a full second of time history to produce a stable and accurate decoder.[57] However, basing motor commands on outdated neural activity reduces responsiveness and negatively affects real-time control. OLE resolves this issue by estimating firing rates based on the previous 450 ms but remains responsive by using an exponential filter to prioritize the most recent samples. Firing rates are collected in 33 ms time bins and input into the OLE to provide velocity predictions. The OLE is calibrated by first modeling the firing rate of each channel as a function of velocities, then finding inverse coefficients for the online decoder. The KF was first introduced in NHP in 2004 and models channel activity as a function of kinematics.[51] This model is then fused with a physical model, reflective of the intended movements, that recursively estimates position and/or velocity states at each time step. Here, the physical model enforces stability, whereas updates to the neural measurement ensure responsiveness. Typical KF implementations execute in intervals ranging from 20 to 100 ms. Both techniques depend on sampling channels that are tuned to different movement directions. Some neurons in the motor cortex may be highly specific to individual movements.[58] However, observing numerous broadly tuned channels may provide sufficient information for control, provided they are well modulated and can be represented by a linear model. In fact, the regularization method in OLE encourages activity from one neuron to be related to more than one kinematic variable. For both the KF and OLE, channels with sparse activity (<1 spike per second average firing rate) during the calibration session are usually ignored. These channels cannot be well represented by linear models, which provide optimal solutions when the predicted variables have normally distributed errors. Neuron spike events closely resemble a Poisson process, which significantly deviates from a normal profile for low firing rates. Evidently, motor prosthetic implementations have succeeded by leveraging profuse channels and large enough processing windows to avoid a problematic violation of this assumption. However, neural interfaces that operate on extremely rapid timescales would benefit from nonlinear techniques.[23]

Following its use in BMI, the KF has been applied to dexterously control multi-DOF hands using inputs from the peripheral motor system. The same framework was successful in both bipolar electrode configurations that measure motor unit activity in specific muscles[16] and referencing schemes that capture potential differences between muscles.[13] However, there are some minor differences between peripheral and BMI implementations. Intracortical electrode grids are designed to interrogate individual neurons in the brain with a high channel count to capture different motor functions. By comparison, intramuscular EMG systems often have lower channel counts but use larger electrodes that capture many nearby motor units. Concerns of sparse activity are therefore not applicable to well-placed EMG leads. Furthermore, because muscles can be individually targeted during surgical implantation,[14–16] engineers can be confident in the functional representation of individual channels. If desired, irrelevant channels can explicitly be masked from decoders instead of relying on automated screening techniques. In the abovementioned clinical studies, the position output of the KF was used to control individual wrist and hand DOF. Velocity control may be useful depending on hardware capabilities, although it is evidently not required. A strong relationship between individual muscles and finger movements produces a decoder that requires less smoothing or active modulation. Patients have used this framework to simultaneously control 3 to 6 wrist and hand DOF using research grade hardware or virtual reality environments.[13,16] The dexterity and precision of control may be limited with commercially available hands that do not offer position or velocity control of individual motors.

BMI and peripheral interfaces can be used to perform different tasks with a variety of end effectors. It is important to consider hardware differences when discussing the limitations of linear regression algorithms. For example, BMI often control computer cursors for communication.[59] In this case, errors may seldom be due to a lack of physical constraints, context changes, and comparatively few DOF. However, for both BMI and peripheral interfaces, directly controlling multi-DOF functional electrical stimulation systems or robotic limbs can prove more challenging. Hardware latency and noise can reduce precision, and a common issue with regression algorithms is the inability to independently activate DOF.[13,52,60] Many reaching and grasping movements use synergistic activations, so this issue may only be apparent for fine motor tasks. In BMI applications, motor neurons are broadly tuned to multiple movements, which can cause problems related to coactivations. Recording from a larger number of neurons theoretically results in better separability of DOF. However, even in EMG applications where specific muscles can easily be targeted, coactivations still cause difficulties for decoders;. This could be due to natural movement synergies required to stabilize joints, which are problematic if they are not properly incorporated into the algorithm. Without a more complete sampling of muscle activity in these contexts, decoders will broadcast these signals as movement commands.

Ultimately, the performance of regression algorithms may be most severely limited by channel count or, in other words, the number of information sources available for each DOF. Techniques to resolve these issues include nonlinear output thresholds[13] and hybrid controllers that use pattern recognition to suppress unwanted activations,[51,61] although these solutions may limit dexterity and increase exertion. Biomechanical models account for natural nonlinearities in muscle activation forces to improve decoder robustness.[62] However, the ability for a hand model to differentiate finger movements depends on the complexity of the model itself as well as muscle synergy mappings in undersampled configurations. Other nonlinear algorithms such as neural networks may one day learn to isolate DOF without sacrificing dexterity.[63] However, approaches with more advanced modeling capabilities may require higher quality calibration data in order to be effective in multiple contexts.[64]

Real-Time Pattern Recognition

Classifiers can be used in to detect movement states or discrete commands in real time. Reducing movement prediction to discrete states can also be useful when there are an insufficient number of channels modulated by a particular movement. In BMI, neural states can be detected to classify hand grasps for FES control.[49] In other implementations, classifiers have been used to improve the performance of virtual cursors by initiating stop or click states.[59,65] The Hidden Markov Model (HMM) has emerged as a common framework to optimize movement state predictions. The HMM represents neural dynamics by explicitly modeling transitions between several underlying latent states.[61] This capability allows the prediction of a click intention, as it occurs in the brain.[59] In addition to stop or click states, classifiers have also been used to suppress unintentional movements of regression controllers by selecting discrete trajectories.[51,61] In this framework, integration delays are extremely costly because they reduce controller responsiveness and the patient's ability to make fine adjustments. Fortunately, the ability of the HMM to model and evaluate state changes over time allows it to operate on rapid timescales without sacrificing stability.[61] In addition to the HMM, deep learning architectures such as recurrent neural networks can recognize temporal dynamics to boost pattern recognition performance of fine motor movements, for example, distinguishing handwritten letters imagined by a patient withSCI.[66] This classifier required characters to be completed before a prediction could be issued, but it demonstrated that complex movements with high temporal variation can be easier to distinguish than less complex gross movements.

Movement classifiers are a natural fit for myoelectric hands that are designed to switch between hand grips rather than individual finger control. Some pattern recognition systems even offer grasp selection capabilities.[5,7,8] However, performance may degrade across different physical contexts.[10] Intramuscular EMG improves controller reliability by providing stable signals with a high signal-to-noise ratio.[15,67] However, it also may allow for techniques such as the HMM to confidently estimate grasp states on faster timescales. Furthermore, access to high resolution muscle signals could increase the number of movements that can be predicted by neural networks.. EMG implementations may differ from BMI in the following ways. For BMI applications, the HMM often characterizes movements with many (up to 20) underlying neural states.[61] To represent downstream muscle activity, only a few latent states may be required per movement. Naive Bayes is commonly used as the latent state model for the HMM because it can model many states without large amounts of training data.[68] However, most BMI implementations have been used for cursor control,[59,65] and myoelectric prostheses need to operate across a wider range of physical contexts. Because intramuscular recordings can provide independent movement signals,[16] it is possible that more robust underlying models can be used without sacrificing predictive power. Similarly, neural networks may be able to predict grasps from EMG with fewer nodes or layers than comparable BMI implementations. Although, as regression algorithms, they may require improvements to the calibration routine.

Calibration Techniques

The performance of both pattern recognition and regression algorithms depends on the quality of calibration data, and this may be especially true for neural networks that may require richer calibration data to take advantage of their increased fitting capabilities.[64] Many research groups use able-bodied participants to validate approaches. Although these volunteers are valuable to the development process, their performance may not directly reflect the capabilities of persons with amputations. A large portion of BMI research is also done with able-bodied NHP. In an able-bodied model, the ground truth of movement intention can be used for training. In that case, ill-fitted parameters can largely be ascribed to a lack of modulated neurons or poorly measured kinematics and motor noise.[69] On the other hand, kinematics cannot easily be measured for patients with injuries or motor system impairments. This can severely limit the quality of training data for fine finger and grasping movements.[64] Neural plasticity may naturally alleviate this issue, as it has been demonstrated that NHP can eventually learn to use BMI with suboptimal parameters.[70] However, advanced calibration techniques can improve performance either by improving initial training data quality or by reducing the learning curve.

Similar to commercial pattern recognition systems, BMI are calibrated by having the user mimic a computer animation or robotic hand to capture neural activity reflective of an intended movement. However, it has been documented that brain activity changes between observed, imagined, and attempted grasps.[71] Patients who lack peripheral motor abilities may have a difficult time consciously distinguishing between these brain states or precisely following movement cues in part due to broken feedback links. In this sense the quality of training data can depend on a patient's sensorimotor function. BMI researchers have found that training grasps with objects in place can improve decoder performance, possibly by encouraging consistent engagement of motor pathways.[56,72] To account for variations in attempted movement speeds, time warping techniques may prove useful by structurally aligning training data.[66] For myoelectric prostheses control, these upstream phenomena could manifest themselves in the improvements noticed with bilateral mirror training.[64]

In cases where an initial training dataset proves difficult to obtain, adaptive calibration techniques have proved effective for BMI. Adaptive calibration for regression algorithms can be completed in single or multiple stages and has shown effective double performance in virtual tasks for arm movements.[21–23] These techniques use goal-oriented supervised tasks, so online control errors and the intended movement can easily be identified and used to reweight parameters. Unsupervised calibration may seem more convenient but requires a framework to automatically identify grasp errors.[73] Supervised techniques may also be preferred to focus on difficult movements and decrease adaptation time.[74] Most supervised approaches estimate the correct movement intention by rotating or aligning the velocity vector toward the goal.[21,22] Finger movements have a short range of motion, and motor cortex hand region neural activity has been shown to be strongly correlated with position as well as velocity. Although it is unclear if existing techniques provide an optimal intention estimate for grasp recalibration, they are still beneficial for BMI.[52] Closed-loop adaptation allows the decoder to recognize shifts in neural tuning between offline calibration and online control.[69] Users also adapt their own behavior to improve online performance of both BMI and EMG controlled devices.[74–76] For BMI, neuroplasticity may play a more prolonged role, reshaping activation patterns to best utilize a given decoder.[76] This type of motor learning is being explored for prosthetic and movement rehabilitation applications even though remapping muscle synergies may be difficult.[77–79] It is unknown how transferrable adaptive BMI techniques will be, as they are only recently being investigated.[74] The success of different calibration techniques for persons with amputations is likely to be individual. Advanced or adaptive calibration methods may not be required for skilled patients who also have excellent perception of their phantom limb but may be increasingly valuable for patients with more proximal or bilateral amputations.

SUMMARY

Intracortical BMI and implantable EMG technologies aim to provide fast and fluid control of upper-limb prostheses by interrogating motor neurons and peripheral motor units, respectively. These high-resolution signals can be fed into high-speed pattern recognition and regression algorithms to control digital cursors or robotic hands. Common solutions may exist to common issues such as unintended movement coactivations or collecting quality calibration data. In the future, BMI may be a rich source of algorithm inspiration, as the number of peripheral channels for EMG systems increases or stable nerve monitoring techniques are developed. Peripheral nerve interfaces may increase the appeal of myoelectric prostheses to patients with more proximal amputations. For patients with varying skill levels and sensorimotor function, enhanced and adaptive calibration techniques can reduce training time

and may be essential to delivering high-performance prosthetic systems.

CLINICS CARE POINTS

- Brain machine interfaces allow patients to fluidly control robotic arms or reanimate previously paralyzed limbs.

- Implantable EMG systems can use similar algorithms to provide dexterous grasp control, although simultaneous and independent control of high DOF systems remain challenging.

- Software solutions are likely to be shared between these 2 technologies, although researchers and engineers must keep in mind some differences.

- Fully implantable electronic systems need to be developed to move both technologies from research to clinic.

REFERENCES

1. Resnik L, Klinger SL, Etter K. The DEKA Arm: its features, functionality, and evolution during the veterans affairs study to optimize the DEKA Arm. Prosthet Orthot Int 2014. https://doi.org/10.1177/0309364613506913.

2. Atzori M, Müller H. Control capabilities of myoelectric robotic prostheses by hand amputees: a scientific research and market overview. Front Syst Neurosci 2015. https://doi.org/10.3389/fnsys.2015.00162.

3. Akhtar A, Choi KY, Fatina M, et al. A low-cost, open-source, compliant hand for enabling sensorimotor control for people with transradial amputations. In: Proceedings of the annual international conference of the IEEE engineering in medicine and biology society, EMBS. 2016. https://doi.org/10.1109/EMBC.2016.7591762.

4. Kuiken TA, Li G, Lock BA, et al. Targeted muscle reinnervation for real-time myoelectric control of multifunction artificial arms. JAMA 2009. https://doi.org/10.1001/jama.2009.116.

5. Kuiken TA, Miller LA, Turner K, et al. A comparison of pattern recognition control and direct control of a multiple degree-of-freedom transradial prosthesis. IEEE J Transl Eng Heal Med 2016. https://doi.org/10.1109/JTEHM.2016.2616123.

6. Cheesborough JE, Smith LH, Kuiken TA, et al. Targeted muscle reinnervation and advanced prosthetic arms. Semin Plast Surg 2015. https://doi.org/10.1055/s-0035-1544166.

7. Kanitz G, Cipriani C, Edin BB. Classification of transient myoelectric signals for the control of multi-grasp hand prostheses. IEEE Trans Neural Syst Rehabil Eng 2018. https://doi.org/10.1109/TNSRE.2018.2861465.

8. Krasoulis A, Vijayakumar S, Nazarpour K. Multi-grip classification-based prosthesis control with two EMG-IMU sensors. IEEE Trans Neural Syst Rehabil Eng 2020. https://doi.org/10.1109/TNSRE.2019.2959243.

9. Farina e D, Vujaklija I, Sartori M, et al. Man/machine interface based on the discharge timings of spinal motor neurons after targeted muscle reinnervation. Nat Biomed Eng 2017;1. https://doi.org/10.1038/s41551-016-0025.

10. Betthauser JL, Hunt CL, Osborn LE, et al. Limb Position Tolerant Pattern Recognition for Myoelectric Prosthesis Control with Adaptive Sparse Representations from Extreme Learning. IEEE Trans Biomed Eng 2018. https://doi.org/10.1109/TBME.2017.2719400.

11. Young AJ, Smith LH, Rouse EJ, et al. Classification of simultaneous movements using surface EMG pattern recognition. IEEE Trans Biomed Eng 2013. https://doi.org/10.1109/TBME.2012.2232293.

12. Engdahl SM, Christie BP, Kelly B, et al. Surveying the interest of individuals with upper limb loss in novel prosthetic control techniques. J Neuroeng Rehabil 2015. https://doi.org/10.1186/s12984-015-0044-2.

13. George JA, Brinton MR, Duncan CC, et al. Improved training paradigms and motor-decode algorithms: results from intact individuals and a recent transradial amputee with prior complex regional pain syndrome. Proc Annu Int Conf IEEE Eng Med Biol Soc EMBS 2018;2018:3782–7.

14. Dewald HA, Lukyanenko P, Lambrecht JM, et al. Stable, three degree-of-freedom myoelectric prosthetic control via chronic bipolar intramuscular electrodes: A case study. J Neuroeng Rehabil 2019. https://doi.org/10.1186/s12984-019-0607-8.

15. Salminger S, Sturma A, Hofer C, et al. Long-term implant of intramuscular sensors and nerve transfers for wireless control of robotic arms in above-elbow amputees. Sci Robot 2019. https://doi.org/10.1126/scirobotics.aaw6306.

16. Vu PP, Vaskov AK, Irwin ZT, et al. A regenerative peripheral nerve interface allows real-time control of an artificial hand in upper limb amputees. Sci Transl Med 2020. https://doi.org/10.1126/scitranslmed.aay2857.

17. Nunez PL, Srinivasan R. Electric fields of the Brain: the Neurophysics of EEG abstract and keywords 1 A window on the mind. Oxford, UK: Oxford University Press; 2006.

18. Nunez PL. Methods to improve spatial resolution of EEG. In: IEEE/Engineering in medicine and biology society annual conference. 1988. https://doi.org/10.1109/iembs.1988.95290.

19. Blabe CH, Gilja V, Chestek CA. Assessment of brain – machine interfaces from the perspective of people with paralysis assessment of brain – machine interfaces from the perspective of people with paralysis. J Neural Eng 2015;12(4):43002.

20. Lahr J, Schwartz C, Heimbach B, et al. Invasive brain-machine interfaces: a survey of paralyzed patients' attitudes, knowledge and methods of information retrieval. J Neural Eng 2015. https://doi.org/10.1088/1741-2560/12/4/043001.

21. Gilja V, Nuyujukian P, Chestek CA, et al. A high-performance neural prosthesis enabled by control algorithm design. Nat Neurosci 2012;15(12):1752–7.

22. Collinger JL, Wodlinger B, Downey JE, et al. High-performance neuroprosthetic control by an individual with tetraplegia. Lancet 2013;381(9866):557–64.

23. Shanechi MM, Orsborn AL, Moorman HG, et al. Rapid control and feedback rates enhance neuroprosthetic control. Nat Commun 2017;8:1–10.

24. Perel S, Sadtler PT, Godlove JM, et al. Direction and speed tuning of motor-cortex multi-unit activity and local field potentials during reaching movements. In: Proceedings of the annual international conference of the IEEE engineering in medicine and biology society, EMBS. 2013. https://doi.org/10.1109/EMBC.2013.6609496.

25. Kennedy SD, Schwartz AB. Distributed processing of movement signaling. Proc Natl Acad Sci U S A 2019. https://doi.org/10.1073/pnas.1902296116.

26. Todorova S, Sadtler P, Batista A, et al. To sort or not to sort: The impact of spike-sorting on neural decoding performance. J Neural Eng 2014. https://doi.org/10.1088/1741-2560/11/5/056005.

27. Fraser GW, Chase SM, Whitford A, et al. Control of a brain-computer interface without spike sorting. J Neural Eng 2009. https://doi.org/10.1088/1741-2560/6/5/055004.

28. Christie BP, Tat DM, Irwin ZT, et al. Comparison of spike sorting and thresholding of voltage waveforms for intracortical brain-machine interface performance. J Neural Eng 2015;12(1):16009. https://doi.org/10.1088/1741-2560/12/1/016009.

29. Stark E, Abeles M. Predicting movement from multiunit activity. J Neurosci 2007. https://doi.org/10.1523/JNEUROSCI.1321-07.2007.

30. Irwin ZT, Thompson DE, Schroeder KE, et al. Enabling low-power, multi-modal neural interfaces through a common, low-bandwidth feature space. IEEE Trans Neural Syst Rehabil Eng 2016. https://doi.org/10.1109/TNSRE.2015.2501752.

31. Nason SR, Vaskov AK, Willsey MS, et al. A low-power band of neuronal spiking activity dominated by local single units improves the performance of brain–machine interfaces. Nat Biomed Eng 2020. https://doi.org/10.1038/s41551-020-0591-0.

32. Flint RD, Wright ZA, Scheid MR, et al. Long term, stable brain machine interface performance using

local field potentials and multiunit spikes. J Neural Eng 2013. https://doi.org/10.1088/1741-2560/10/5/056005.

33. Stavisky SD, Kao JC, Nuyujukian P, et al. A high performing brain-machine interface driven by low-frequency local field potentials alone and together with spikes. J Neural Eng 2015. https://doi.org/10.1088/1741-2560/12/3/036009.

34. Jackson A, Hall TM. Decoding local field potentials for neural interfaces. IEEE Trans Neural Syst Rehabil Eng 2017. https://doi.org/10.1109/TNSRE.2016.2612001.

35. Suner S, Fellows MR, Vargas-Irwin C, et al. Reliability of signals from a chronically implanted, silicon-based electrode array in non-human primate primary motor cortex. IEEE Trans Neural Syst Rehabil Eng 2005. https://doi.org/10.1109/TNSRE.2005.857687.

36. Simeral JD, Kim SP, Black MJ, et al. Neural control of cursor trajectory and click by a human with tetraplegia 1000 days after implant of an intracortical microelectrode array. J Neural Eng 2011;8(2):25027.

37. Chestek CA, Gilja V, Nuyujukian P, et al. Long-term stability of neural prosthetic control signals from silicon cortical arrays in rhesus macaque motor cortex. J Neural Eng 2011. https://doi.org/10.1088/1741-2560/8/4/045005.

38. Patel PR, Zhang H, Robbins MT, et al. Chronic in vivo stability assessment of carbon fiber microelectrode arrays. J Neural Eng 2016. https://doi.org/10.1088/1741-2560/13/6/066002.

39. Welle EJ, Patel PR, Woods JE, et al. Ultra-small carbon fiber electrode recording site optimization and improved in vivo chronic recording yield. J Neural Eng 2020. https://doi.org/10.1088/1741-2552/ab8343.

40. Guido K, Clavijo A, Zhu K, et al. Strategies to Improve Neural Electrode Performance. Neural Interf Eng 2020. https://doi.org/10.1007/978-3-030-41854-0_7.

41. Volkova K, Lebedev MA, Kaplan A, et al. Decoding movement from electrocorticographic activity: a review. Front Neuroinform 2019. https://doi.org/10.3389/fninf.2019.00074.

42. Vansteensel MJ, Pels EGM, Bleichner MG, et al. Fully implanted brain–computer interface in a locked-in patient with ALS. N Engl J Med 2016. https://doi.org/10.1056/nejmoa1608085.

43. Bullard AJ, Nason SR, Irwin ZT, et al. Design and testing of a 96-channel neural interface module for the Networked Neuroprosthesis system. Bioelectron Med 2019. https://doi.org/10.1186/s42234-019-0019-x.

44. Wang PT, Camacho E, Wang M, et al. A benchtop system to assess the feasibility of a fully independent and implantable brain-machine interface. J Neural Eng 2019. https://doi.org/10.1088/1741-2552/ab4b0c.

45. Benabid AL, Costecalde T, Eliseyev A, et al. An exoskeleton controlled by an epidural wireless brain–machine interface in a tetraplegic patient: a proof-of-concept demonstration. Lancet Neurol 2019. https://doi.org/10.1016/S1474-4422(19)30321-7.

46. Weir RF, Troyk PR, DeMichele GA, et al. Implantable myoelectric sensors (IMESs) for intramuscular electromyogram recording. IEEE Trans Biomed Eng 2009. https://doi.org/10.1109/TBME.2008.2005942.

47. Santosa KB, Oliver JD, Cederna PS, et al. Regenerative peripheral nerve interfaces for prevention and management of neuromas. Clin Plast Surg 2020. https://doi.org/10.1016/j.cps.2020.01.004.

48. Ajiboye AB, Willett FR, Young DR, et al. Restoration of reaching and grasping movements through brain-controlled muscle stimulation in a person with tetraplegia: a proof-of-concept demonstration. Lancet 2017;389(10081):1821–30. https://doi.org/10.1016/S0140-6736(17)30601-3.

49. Colachis SC, Bockbrader MA, Zhang M, et al. Dexterous control of seven functional hand movements using cortically-controlled transcutaneous muscle stimulation in a person with tetraplegia. Front Neurosci 2018;12(APR):208. https://doi.org/10.3389/fnins.2018.00208.

50. Hochberg LR, Bacher D, Jarosiewicz B, et al. Reach and grasp by people with tetraplegia using a neurally controlled robotic arm. Nature 2012;485(7398):372–5. https://doi.org/10.1038/nature11076.

51. Wu W, Black MJ, Mumford D, et al. Modeling and decoding motor cortical activity using a switching Kalman filter. IEEE Trans Biomed Eng 2004. https://doi.org/10.1109/TBME.2004.826666.

52. Vaskov AK, Irwin ZT, Nason SR, et al. Cortical decoding of individual finger group motions using ReFIT Kalman filter. Front Neurosci 2018;12:751. https://doi.org/10.3389/fnins.2018.00751.

53. Marathe AR, Taylor DM. Decoding position, velocity, or goal: does it matter for brain-machine interfaces? J Neural Eng 2011. https://doi.org/10.1088/1741-2560/8/2/025016.

54. Zhang Y, Chase SM. Recasting brain-machine interface design from a physical control system perspective. J Comput Neurosci 2015. https://doi.org/10.1007/s10827-015-0566-4.

55. Cunningham JP, Nuyujukian P, Gilja V, et al. A closed-loop human simulator for investigating the role of feedback control in brain-machine interfaces. J Neurophysiol 2011;105(4):1932–49.

56. Wodlinger B, Downey JE, Tyler-Kabara EC, et al. Ten-dimensional anthropomorphic arm control in a human brain-machine interface: difficulties, solutions, and limitations. J Neural Eng 2015;12(1):16011.

57. Serruya MD, Hatsopoulos NG, Paninski L, et al. Brain-machine interface: Instant neural control of a

movement signal. Nature 2002;416(6877):141–2. https://doi.org/10.1038/416141a.

58. Aggarwal V, Acharya S, Tenore F, et al. Asynchronous decoding of dexterous finger movements using M1 neurons. IEEE Trans Neural Syst Rehabil Eng 2008;16(1):3–14.

59. Pandarinath C, Nuyujukian P, Blabe CH, et al. High performance communication by people with paralysis using an intracortical brain-computer interface. Elife 2017;6:18554.

60. Hahne JM, Schweisfurth MA, Koppe M, et al. Simultaneous control of multiple functions of bionic hand prostheses: performance and robustness in end users. Sci Robot 2018. https://doi.org/10.1126/scirobotics.aat3630.

61. Kemere C, Santhanam G, Yu BM, et al. Neural-state transitions using hidden markov models for motor cortical prostheses. J Neurophysiol 2008;100: 2441–52.

62. Sartori M, Durandau G, Došen S, et al. Robust simultaneous myoelectric control of multiple degrees of freedom in wrist-hand prostheses by real-time neuromusculoskeletal modeling. J Neural Eng 2018. https://doi.org/10.1088/1741-2552/aae26b.

63. Dantas H, Warren DJ, Wendelken S, et al. Deep learning movement intent decoders trained with dataset aggregation for prosthetic limb control. IEEE Trans Biomed Eng 2019;66(11):3192–202.

64. George JA, Tully TN, Colgan PC, et al. Bilaterally mirrored movements improve the accuracy and precision of training data for supervised learning of neural or myoelectric prosthetic control. In: Proceedings of the annual international conference of the IEEE engineering in medicine and biology society, EMBS. 2020. https://doi.org/10.1109/EMBC44109.2020.9175388.

65. Kao JC, Nuyujukian P, Ryu SI, et al. A high-performance neural prosthesis incorporating discrete state selection with hidden markov models. IEEE Trans Biomed Eng 2017. https://doi.org/10.1109/TBME.2016.2582691.

66. Willett FR, Avansino DT, Hochberg LR, et al. High-performance brain-to-text communication via handwriting. Nature 2021;593(7858). https://doi.org/10.1038/s41586-021-03506-2.

67. OrtizCatalan M, Mastinu E, Sassu P, et al. Self-contained neuromusculoskeletal arm prostheses. N Engl J Med 2020. https://doi.org/10.1056/NEJMoa1917537.

68. Domingos P, Pazzani M. On the Optimality of the simple bayesian classifier under zero-one loss.

Mach Learn 1997. https://doi.org/10.1023/A:1007413511361.

69. Fan JM, Nuyujukian P, Kao JC, et al. Intention estimation in brain-machine interfaces. J Neural Eng 2014;11(1):16004.

70. Heliot R, Ganguly K, Carmena JM. Modeling and experimental validation of the learning process during closed-loop bmi operation. In: Proceedings of the 2009 international conference on machine learning and cybernetics. 2009. https://doi.org/10.1109/ICMLC.2009.5212798.

71. Rastogi A, Vargas-Irwin CE, Willett FR, et al. Neural Representation of Observed, Imagined, and Attempted Grasping Force in Motor Cortex of Individuals with Chronic Tetraplegia. Sci Rep 2020. https://doi.org/10.1038/s41598-020-58097-1.

72. Downey JE, Brane L, Gaunt RA, et al. Motor cortical activity changes during neuroprosthetic-controlled object interaction. Sci Rep 2017. https://doi.org/10.1038/s41598-017-17222-3.

73. Meattini R, Nowak M, Melchiorri C, et al. Automated instability detection for interactive myocontrol of prosthetic hands. Front Neurorobot 2019. https://doi.org/10.3389/fnbot.2019.00068.

74. Couraud M, Cattaert D, Paclet F, et al. Model and experiments to optimize co-adaptation in a simplified myoelectric control system. J Neural Eng 2018. https://doi.org/10.1088/1741-2552/aa87cf.

75. Krasoulis A, Vijayakumar S, Nazarpour K. Effect of user practice on prosthetic finger control with an intuitive myoelectric decoder. Front Neurosci 2019. https://doi.org/10.3389/fnins.2019.00891.

76. Oby ER, Golub MD, Hennig JA, et al. New neural activity patterns emerge with long-term learning. Proc Natl Acad Sci U S A 2019. https://doi.org/10.1073/pnas.1820296116.

77. Barnes J, Dyson M, Nazarpour K. Comparison of hand and forearm muscle pairs in controlling of a novel myoelectric interface. In: 2016 IEEE international conference on systems, man, and cybernetics, SMC 2016 - conference Proceedings. 2017. https://doi.org/10.1109/SMC.2016.7844671.

78. Pierella C, Abdollahi F, Farshchiansadegh A, et al. Remapping residual coordination for controlling assistive devices and recovering motor functions. Neuropsychologia 2015. https://doi.org/10.1016/j.neuropsychologia.2015.08.024.

79. Berger DJ, Gentner R, Edmunds T, et al. Differences in adaptation rates after virtual surgeries provide direct evidence for modularity. J Neurosci 2013. https://doi.org/10.1523/JNEUROSCI.0122-13.2013.

Fascicle-Specific Targeting of Longitudinal Intrafascicular Electrodes for Motor and Sensory Restoration in Upper-Limb Amputees

Jonathan Cheng, MD[a],*, Zhi Yang, PhD[b], Cynthia K. Overstreet, PhD[c], Edward Keefer, PhD[c]

KEYWORDS

- Peripheral nerve • Electrical stimulation • Prosthetic control • Motor decoding • Machine learning
- Fascicle • Amputee

KEY POINTS

- Fascicle-specific targeting (FAST) of longitudinal intrafascicular electrodes (LIFE), also known as FAST-LIFE electrode interfacing, is a surgical strategy for placing neural interfaces within the discrete sensory- and motor-related fascicular groups of the residual peripheral nerves in upper limb amputees.
- FAST-LIFE interfacing permits selectivity of electrical stimulation to restore touch and movement-associated sensations.
- Used together with custom electronics for recording peripheral nerve signals and artificial intelligence decoding of motor intent, FAST-LIFE interfacing provides motor control signals sufficient to command individual digit motion of a robotic hand prosthesis.
- FAST-LIFE electrode interfacing enables motor and sensory restoration for multiple levels of upper limb amputation and can be performed decades after injury.
- FAST-LIFE interfacing for sensory stimulation and motor recording/decoding holds promise as a research tool and clinical modality for central nervous system and peripheral nervous system disorders impacting motor control of intact and injured limbs.

 Video content accompanies this article at http://www.hand.theclinics.com.

INTRODUCTION

Advances in the engineering of robotic limbs have resulted in hand/upper extremity prostheses with near-anatomic weight and size, and up to 26 degrees of freedom (DoF) of movement.[1] Despite this important progress, the uptake and continued use of robotic prostheses by upper limb amputees remain disappointing. Abandonment of robotic prostheses by users is reported to be as high as 50% in some studies.[2]

The poor acceptance of robotic limb prostheses by upper limb amputees has been attributed

[a] Department of Plastic Surgery, University of Texas Southwestern Medical Center, 1801 Inwood Road, Dallas, TX 75390, USA; [b] Department of Biomedical Engineering, University of Minnesota, Nils Hasselmo Hall, Room 6-120, 312 Church Street Southeast, Minneapolis, MN 55455, USA; [c] Nerves Incorporated, P.O. Box 141295, Dallas, TX 75214, USA
* Corresponding author.
E-mail address: jonathan.cheng@utsouthwestern.edu

Hand Clin 37 (2021) 401–414
https://doi.org/10.1016/j.hcl.2021.04.004
0749-0712/21/© 2021 Elsevier Inc. All rights reserved.

to poor utility and embodiment, because of limitations in the interface between the robotic prosthesis and its user. Specifically, current state-of-the-art prosthetic control interfaces rely on muscle-based signals, which use the residual forearm muscles to control gross motions, including forearm rotation, wrist flexion/extension, and digit flexion/extension. Importantly, muscle-based prosthetic control cannot afford independent digit control for a variety of reasons related to the anatomy and physiology of the amputation stump. Furthermore, existing robotic prostheses do not provide feedback to the user in the form of naturalistic tactile, kinesthetic, and proprioceptive sensations.

To address these limitations, we have devised *fascicle-specific targeting (FAST) of longitudinal intrafascicular electrodes (LIFE)*, also known as FAST-LIFE electrode interfacing. This strategy is a peripheral nerve-centered interfacing strategy for the delivery of 2 key factors, independent digit control and physiologically congruent sensory feedback, to provide users with "dexterous" robotic hand control. FAST-LIFE electrode interfacing surgically targets neural interfaces to the discrete sensory- and motor-related fascicular groups of residual peripheral nerves in upper limb amputees[3] (**Fig. 1**).

FASCICLE-SPECIFIC TARGETING OF LONGITUDINAL INTRAFASCICULAR ELECTRODES

In FAST-LIFE electrode interfacing, microsurgical dissection is performed on the residual ulnar and median nerve trunks of the amputated limb in order to identify and separate the motor and sensory fascicular groups located within the nerves. Intraneural electrodes are then surgically targeted to these fascicular groups, providing access to the sensory- and motor-related functions located in the constituent axons of each fascicle. This microsurgical approach was motivated by the primary author's (J.C.) clinical practice in peripheral nerve reconstruction, where nerve transfers are used at all levels of the brachial plexus for restoration of missing functions (**Fig. 2**).

Microsurgical dissection of intraneural fascicles is a technique inherent to nerve transfers distal to the midhumeral level. The routine clinical use of nerve transfers has opened the eyes of our research team to the discrete motor and sensory functions available through access of these intraneural fascicles[4–9] (**Table 1**). By specifically interfacing with the sensory fascicles, we are able to selectively stimulate afferent nerve fibers, which provide anatomically localized touch sensation in

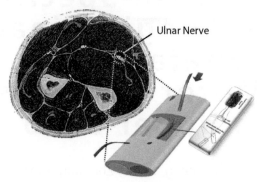

Fig. 1. FAST-LIFE electrode implantation to the ulnar nerve at the forearm, with 1 set of multichannel electrodes targeted directly into each of the microsurgically dissected sensory and motor fascicular groups. The sensory fascicular group (*green*) represents 60% of the nerve cross-sectional area (CSA), and the motor fascicular group (*blue*) represents 40% of the nerve CSA.

the associated cutaneous territories.[3] Surgical targeting of the motor fascicles (deep motor fascicle of ulnar nerve, thenar motor fascicle of median nerve) provides a unique opportunity to selectively stimulate segregated muscle-related afferent nerve fibers for kinesthetic (sensations of movement) and proprioceptive (sensations of force and position) sensory feedback.[3] Finally, FAST-LIFE electrode interfacing of the motor fascicles places electrode contacts directly adjacent to the motor axons carrying control information intended for the small muscles of the hand. These muscles, the ulnar-innervated intrinsic muscles and the median- and ulnar-innervated thenar muscles, participate in every movement of every digit of the intact hand.[10] By recording the motor control signals

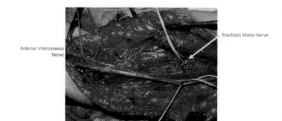

Fig. 2. Clinical example of microsurgical intraneural dissection of a motor fascicle for nerve transfer. The anterior interosseous nerve (*red loop*) has been dissected from the proximal forearm to the midhumeral level, to prepare it as the recipient nerve for a transfer of the brachialis motor nerve (*blue loop*). The biceps has been reflected laterally. This transfer is used to reconstruct grasp/pinch function in lower trunk brachial plexus palsy patients with an otherwise paralyzed hand.

Table 1
Sensory and motor fascicular groups of the ulnar and median nerves provide access to specific sensory and motor functions

	Sensory Fascicles	Motor Fascicles
Ulnar nerve	Touch and joint movement sensation for small finger and ulnar half of ring finger	Kinesthetic and proprioceptive sensation for all digits Motor control for intrinsic muscles and many thenar muscles
Median nerve	Touch and joint movement sensation for thumb, index, long fingers, and radial half of ring finger	Kinesthetic and proprioceptive sensation for thumb, index, long fingers Motor control for thenar muscles, lumbricals of index and long fingers

intended for the elements of the hand that are absent in upper limb amputees, we have gained sufficient motor control data to command individual finger movements of a robotic hand prosthesis.[11]

TARGET POPULATIONS
Partial Hand Amputees

Partial hand amputation patients are missing most of their fingers and possibly their thumb (**Fig. 3**). The partial hand level constitutes the highest proportion of upper limb amputations, accounting for ~90%.[12] Despite the predominance of the partial hand amputation level, this patient population is relatively underserved by existing robotic hand prostheses because of the following: high variability of anatomic presentations obviating standardized off-the-shelf prosthetics, and lack of sensory feedback and individual digit control in commercially available customizable, modular robotic hand systems suitable for partial hand restoration.[13] These patients typically prefer to use their native motor function provided by the residual carpus, metacarpals, and any remaining digits, over the awkward artificial grasp patterns provided by a robotic partial hand prosthesis. They also have stringent design needs for prosthetic fitting and anchoring, as any prosthetic worn on the hand can easily "blind" their critical remaining hand sensation and becomes a barrier to its routine use.

In the United States alone, there are ~17,000 new partial hand amputees per year, indicating a substantial patient population with an inadequately addressed need for prosthetic rehabilitation.[14] In this study, we have investigated the application of peripheral nerve interfacing for prosthetic control in partial hand amputees for the first time. By providing sensory feedback from the prosthetic digits and motor commands to control the individual digits of a customizable modular robotic hand prosthesis, FAST-LIFE electrode interfacing holds promise for addressing the critical deficits that currently exist in prosthetic hand rehabilitation for partial hand amputees.

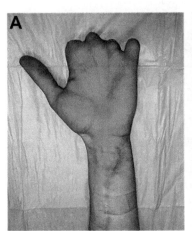
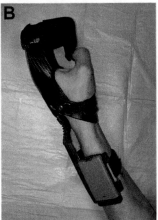

Fig. 3. (A) Partial hand amputation with absent fingers and preserved thumb, in a 24-year-old man with injury sustained 9 months before while using an industrial press. (B) Partial hand amputee wearing custom modular robotic partial hand prosthesis, controlled using surface EMG signals from the extrinsic forearm muscles. This prosthesis does not provide naturalistic sensory feedback.

Transradial Amputees

Transradial, or forearm-level, amputees (**Fig. 4**) constitute the greatest focus of upper limb robotic prosthesis technology development. This focus is driven by the availability of retained forearm muscles in most patients with amputations distal to the proximal third of the forearm. Myoelectric hands, which are robotic hand prostheses controlled using surface electromyogram (EMG) signals from the residual forearm muscles, are produced by at least 7 different commercial manufacturers at the time of this publication. Because of inadequate control mechanisms and lack of sensorization, these myoelectric hand systems are not able to provide naturalistic sensory feedback or individual digit control in routine clinical practice. The absence of sensation and individual digit control leads to a lack of robotic hand dexterity and contributes directly to the abandonment of robotic hand prostheses by up to 50% of transradial amputees.[2] Developing the relevant scientific understanding and a unified technical approach to address these unmet needs is a primary focus of our research team's work.

Transhumeral and Glenohumeral Amputees (Future)

Our future work will expand FAST-LIFE electrode interfacing to experimental clinical studies on patients with transhumeral and glenohumeral amputations. Although the deep motor fascicle of the ulnar nerve and the thenar motor fascicle of the median nerve are not present at these more proximal levels, the medial cord and lateral cord contributions to the median nerve provide a convenient anatomic site where sensory and motor axons are segregated into discrete fascicles and available for FAST-LIFE targeting. At these levels, the ulnar nerve also contains discrete intraneural fascicles[15] that can be individually targeted with FAST-LIFE electrodes to provide high channel counts for high DoF prosthetic control and functional redundancy for long-term interfacing robustness.

Conventional and experimental approaches that use EMG of the forearm or hand muscles for myoelectric prosthesis control obviously cannot be used alone at the transhumeral and glenohumeral levels, because of the total absence of the muscles that would supply EMG control signals. Targeted muscle reinnervation (TMR) surgery can provide some degree of myoelectric hand control for transhumeral and glenohumeral amputees, but TMR has provided neither naturalistic sensory feedback nor individual digit control to date and may represent a long-term detriment to the patient by obviating the future use of promising nerve-only interfacing strategies.[16] By using nerve-only interfacing for both sensory feedback and motor control, FAST-LIFE electrode interfacing presents a unique potential opportunity for dexterous robotic hand restoration in these highly impaired proximal amputees.

CASE SERIES

All clinical studies described in this article were approved by the University of Texas Southwestern Medical Center Institutional Review Board (IRB) as well as the Department of the Navy, Human Research Protection Office.

We performed 3 partial hand and 3 transradial FAST-LIFE electrode implantation trials, as part of the DARPA Hand Proprioceptive and Touch Interfaces (HAPTIX) research program for direct-to-clinical translation. Implant duration ranged from 3 to 16 months and was determined based on

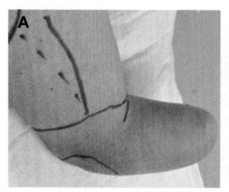
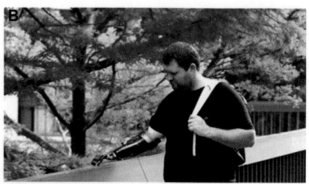

Fig. 4. (*A*) Transradial amputee (male, 31 years old) with mid-forearm level of amputation sustained 3 years before while using an industrial press. (*B*) Transradial amputee wearing a research myoelectric hand fitted with touch sensors, attached to his existing home prosthetic socket for anchoring to his residual forearm. The touch sensors cue electrical stimulation of the ulnar and median nerves to provide tactile sensory feedback during use of the robotic hand.

the increasing maximum time permitted by the IRB over the course of our study and each patient's participation. Patients came to the laboratory as frequently as once a week for electrophysiology and prosthetic control experiments, beginning the week after implantation. Explantation surgery was performed at the conclusion of the patient's participation in the trial.

Patient ages were 52, 58, 44, 21, 32, and 46 years; time elapsed since amputation was 20 years, 11 years, 7 years, 9 months, 4 years, 10 years, respectively. FAST-LIFE interfacing of the residual ulnar nerve was successful in all partial hand patients, and of the residual ulnar and median nerves in all transradial patients. No patients had increased pain beyond the immediate postoperative period, and no patients suffered permanent functional impairment as a result of their participation in these trials. One partial hand and 1 transradial patient had lasting relief of preexisting neuropathic pain as a result of their FAST-LIFE implantation surgery, likely because of surgical release of nerve compression sites identified during their procedures.

PREOPERATIVE ASSESSMENT
Physical Examination

All patients were examined to confirm that strength and sensation of the residual limb, skin condition, joint mobility, vascularity, pain/tenderness, edema, amputation stump quality, and condition and function of residual digits/limb are suitable for participation.

Plain Radiographs

Radiographs were reviewed for bony anatomy of the amputation stump, suitability for electrode implants, and future fitting of prosthetics. This review also provided a baseline examination for tracking the postoperative appearance of the limb and implants using radiographs.

Magnetic Resonance Neurography

Magnetic resonance neurography (MRN) was performed to detail the location and condition of amputated peripheral nerve stumps in the residual limb, because the external appearance of the amputation stump often does not correspond to the injury level of internal structures depending on the nature of the original injury (eg, sharp transection vs avulsion). The MRN also provides the surgeon with information regarding the innervation status and anatomic configuration of residual forearm/hand muscles, which is relevant to the placement and function of planned FAST-LIFE electrodes. On 2 patients, 1 partial hand and 1 transradial, MRN revealed preexisting compression neuropathy in the residual limb, which was surgically released during the process of FAST-LIFE electrode implantation.

Electrodiagnostic Studies

Nerve conduction studies (NCS) were performed to assess motor and sensory conduction of the median and ulnar nerves, and EMG of the residual forearm and hand muscles was performed to confirm their innervation status. NCS and EMG provide information regarding the health of residual nerves and muscles in the amputated limb, and when abnormal, may reveal residual, lasting dysfunction from the original injury, which could impact the ability to perform FAST-LIFE interfacing.

It is important to note that NCS often cannot provide sufficient assessment of preexisting compression neuropathy within the amputation stump because of the absence of terminal end organs (cutaneous sensory receptors, small hand muscles), which are required for quantitative comparison of recorded values against established norms.[17] These physiologically incomplete sensory and motor neural circuits pose a substantial limitation on the electrodiagnosis of compression neuropathy as a cause of neuropathic pain (eg, residual limb pain vs phantom limb pain) in major limb amputees.

SURGICAL PROCEDURES

All surgery is performed under inhalational general anesthetic in the operating suite. Tourniquets are used for up to 30 minutes at a time to prevent tourniquet-induced nerve palsy and permit nerve stimulator use. Somatosensory-evoked potentials are obtained to provide electrophysiologic differentiation of motor versus sensory nerve fascicles, and a handheld nerve stimulator is used to confirm motor fascicles if distal muscles are present and functioning. The operating microscope is used to perform microdissection of the selected sensory and motor fascicles and to place the intraneural components of the FAST-LIFE electrodes (Video 1).

POSTOPERATIVE CARE

Patients are immobilized in a splint for 3 weeks after implantation surgery, to allow electrodes and wiring positions to stabilize. They begin wear and use of their existing myoelectric prosthesis at 6 weeks after surgery.

MOTOR RECORDING/DECODING

Custom recording electronics were designed by members of our group at the University of

Minnesota, with hardware-based noise and artifact rejection circuitry to permit recording of peripheral nerve-derived motor control signals.[11,18,19] This capability is the linchpin of the motor control strategy in our FAST-LIFE electrode interfacing approach. Peripheral nerve signals are relatively small compared with nerve signals routinely obtained from the brain cortex, and there is substantial noise and movement-related artifact owing to the inherent anatomy of the limbs. The ability to chronically record peripheral nerve signals is a feature unique to FAST-LIFE interfacing, as other peripheral prosthetic control strategies for robotic hands remain centered on muscle-derived signals.

Novel artificial intelligence (AI; machine learning) algorithms are used to decode the motor control signals obtained using FAST-LIFE electrodes, primarily using the electrodes in the targeted motor fascicles.[11] As all of our patients were unilateral amputees with an intact contralateral limb, we were able to initiate development and training of the AI algorithms using a motion tracking glove worn on the contralateral hand while the subject performed identical gestures with both hands. Hand gestures consisted of "imagined" hand movement on the amputated side, and "real" voluntary hand movement on the contralateral intact side. FAST-LIFE motor control signal recordings from the amputated side were processed together with simultaneous "ground truth" motion-tracking data from the intact side to train the AI algorithms. Our AI algorithms delivered reliable decoding of FAST-LIFE motor control signals for up to 17 DoF of hand movement (**Table 2**). Decoding accuracy was estimated at 80% to 90%, based on a VAF (variance accounted for) score of 0.8 to 0.9 (**Fig. 5**). Decoded FAST-LIFE motor control signals were sufficient to command individual movement of all 5 digits on a robotic hand prosthesis (Video 2).

SENSORY STIMULATION

Sensory stimulation was directed toward FAST-LIFE electrodes within the sensory and motor fascicles to selectively elicit tactile versus proprioceptive sensations. In partial hand amputees, FAST-LIFE interfacing was performed with the ulnar nerve motor and sensory fascicles. In transradial amputees, FAST-LIFE interfacing was performed with the median and ulnar nerves, with specific targeting of the motor and sensory fascicles in each nerve trunk. The sensory fascicle FAST-LIFE electrodes yielded sensations in the typical cutaneous distribution of the respective nerve trunk (**Fig. 6**). The motor

| Table 2 |
| Artificial intelligence-based motor decoding algorithms were trained on 17 degrees-of-freedom of upper limb movement |

DoF Indices	Joints/Movements
1	Thumb MP
2	Thumb IP
3	Index MP
4	Index PIP
5	Long MP
6	Long PIP
7	Ring MP
8	Ring PIP
9	Small MP
10	Small PIP
11	Thumb abduction
12	Index abduction
13	Long abduction
14	Ring abduction
15	Thumb opposition
16	Wrist flexion
17	Wrist pronation

Decoding was performed on motor control signals recorded using custom electronics from FAST-LIFE electrodes, with motion-tracking data collected from the contralateral intact limb serving as the "ground truth" training data set.

Abbreviations: DoF, degree-of-freedom; IP, interphalangeal joint; MP, metacarpophalangeal joint; PIP, proximal interphalangeal joint.

fascicles, which include sensory afferents arising from the intrinsic and/or thenar muscles, were used to evoke proprioceptive sensations covering a much broader area of the hand because of the wide anatomic distribution of those muscles (**Fig. 7**).

Sensory stimulation experiments included exploration of a wide variety of stimulation parameters, which we found to permit variation in quality, intensity, location, area, and duration of elicited sensations.[3] Patients were able to reliably discriminate between at least 7 different stimulation intensities, and this could enable a robotic hand user to scale pinch-and-grip force activation during object manipulation using graded tactile sensory feedback. Proprioceptive sensations delivered through the motor fascicles provide the opportunity for "closed loop" motor control of robotic hands by giving the amputee kinesthetic sensory feedback during voluntary movement of the prosthesis.

We also found that body position sense was improved simply by adding functionally congruent

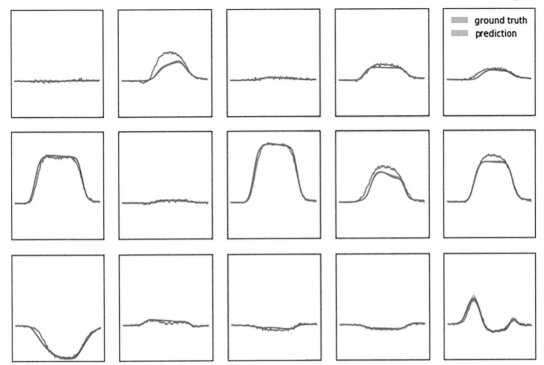

Fig. 5. Individual movement activation predictions (*orange*) using AI decoding of motor control signals recorded from FAST-LIFE electrodes, superimposed upon "ground truth" movement training data (*blue*) collected from a motion tracking glove worn on the contralateral intact limb. Each rectangle represents 1 of the 15 DoF decoded.

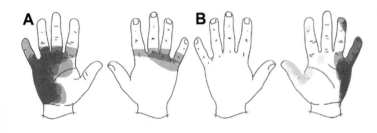

Fig. 6. Electrical stimulation of median and/or ulnar *sensory* fascicles in (*A*) partial hand amputee, (*B*) transradial amputee. Receptive field of ulnar nerve cutaneous sensory percepts (*red*); median nerve cutaneous sensory percepts (*blue*). Intensity of color reflects frequency of receptive field activation by different electrode sites on the multichannel FAST-LIFE implant in each nerve trunk. Evoked sensations included "brushing," "pulsing," "stinging," and "tingling."

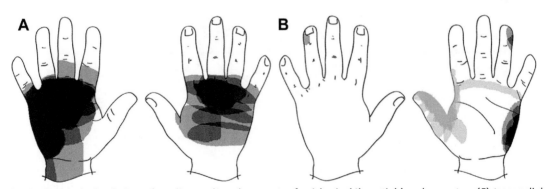

Fig. 7. Electrical stimulation of median and/or ulnar *motor* fascicles in (*A*) partial hand amputee, (*B*) transradial amputee. Receptive field of ulnar nerve proprioceptive sensory percepts (*blue*), median nerve proprioceptive sensory percepts (*green*). Intensity of color reflects frequency of receptive field activation by different electrode sites on the multichannel FAST-LIFE electrode in each nerve trunk. Evoked sensations included "curling," "moving," "squeezing."

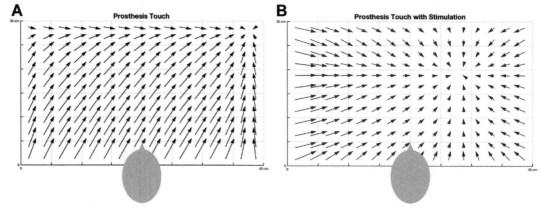

Fig. 8. Body-centered proprioceptive mapping assessment: (*A*) without sensory feedback, (*B*) with functionally congruent sensory feedback. The patient was wearing a standard myoelectric robotic hand prosthesis and was blindfolded while a fingertip was touched to the 2-dimensional surface grid centered on the patient's seated location. Without sensation, their perceived location of the robotic hand was substantially skewed away and toward the side wearing the prosthetic hand. With electrically stimulated fingertip sensation, position sense for the location of the robotic hand was greatly improved.

touch sensation through a single fingertip of a myoelectric robotic hand (**Fig. 8**). Using the proprioceptive mapping assessment described by Rincon-Gonzalez and colleagues,[20] we found that patients using a plain myoelectric robotic hand prosthesis had highly altered proprioception, with substantially skewed perception of where their hand was positioned in space. When tactile sensory feedback was delivered through the FAST-LIFE electrode interface during the proprioceptive mapping assessment, the patient's proprioception was corrected toward normal, and they had an improved ability to perceive the position of their hand with an error reduction of 15% (see **Fig. 8**). This surprising finding hints at the enormous potential value of providing both tactile and proprioceptive sensation during use of a robotic hand. There is likely to be a dynamic interplay between multiple submodality sensory feedback, peripheral nerve-driven motor control, and robotic hand use that is synergistic rather than additive.

Finally, we demonstrated that functional task performance was greatly improved when we added tactile sensory feedback to patients' myoelectric robotic hands. Improved functional task performance was shown during block stacking, cup stacking, and dual tasking functional trials (**Fig. 9**). When sensory feedback was turned on, patients displayed greater persistence in using their myoelectric robotic hand, spending 30% more time exploring or attempting difficult tasks.

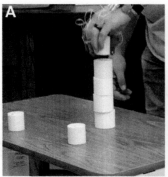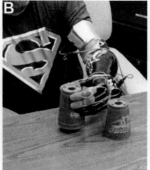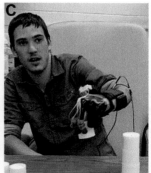

Fig. 9. Functional trials showed improved outcomes when sensory feedback was turned on. (*A*) Basic object manipulation. Time to stack 7 sequentially sized cylindrical blocks was decreased by 20% to 35%. (*B*) Light grasp accuracy. Time to unstack and stack 3 cups was improved by 40% to 70%. (*C*) Cognitive load reduction. The time to complete block stacking task described in panel (A) while simultaneously performing standardized verbal task was reduced by 10% to 14%.

CASE EXAMPLE: PARTIAL HAND (PATIENT 4)

N.B. is a 21-year-old right hand–dominant welder/fabricator. In May 2017, he was involved in a work accident. He was training a new employee on how to use a brake press when his left hand was crushed within the press. He had an initial 12-hour reconstruction of his fingers, but ultimately had amputation of all his fingers at the proximal phalanx level in June 2017 (see **Fig. 3**). A Touch Bionics myoelectric robotic partial hand serves as his primary prosthesis, which he uses at home and at work.

His nondominant hand was amputated at the proximal shaft of the proximal phalanges in all fingers, although his thumb was preserved and functioning (**Fig. 10**). MRN revealed increased signal of the median and ulnar nerves in the forearm, with findings suggestive of mild carpal tunnel syndrome. The patient reported no symptoms of carpal tunnel syndrome, and these MRN changes were attributed to the traumatic injury (**Fig. 11**). EMG showed polyphasic action potentials in the first dorsal interosseous muscle, likely because of local trauma in the hand (**Fig. 12**).

Multichannel FAST-LIFE electrodes were implanted to the motor and sensory fascicular groups of the ulnar nerve at the distal forearm. There were 15 data channels per electrode, for a total of 30 channels. Wires from the FAST-LIFE electrodes were passed through the skin of the volar forearm and terminated in an external connector block (**Fig. 13**).

The patient was seen in our laboratory at UT Southwestern for experimental sessions weekly, beginning the week after implantation surgery. Electrical stimulation of the sensory and motor fascicles of the ulnar nerve evoked tactile and proprioceptive sensations in the related anatomic territories, with sensory fascicle receptive fields confined to the ring and small finger axes and motor fascicle receptive fields spread out over the hand where intrinsic and thenar muscles are located (**Fig. 14**).

Motor recording and decoder training were performed during 2 sessions with this patient (**Fig. 15**). However, he was involved in a motorcycle accident during his participation in this clinical trial and was ultimately explanted because of this at 5 months after implantation. He has returned to normal use of his existing custom myoelectric partial hand prosthesis made with modular components for his specific anatomy (see **Fig. 3**), without any functional effects from his participation in this trial.

CASE EXAMPLE: TRANSRADIAL (PATIENT 5)

C.S. is a 32-year-old right hand–dominant machinist. He suffered a right transradial amputation 3 years before, when he was using a machine press at an oilfield services company. His initial care was at Parkland Memorial Hospital, our university's level 1 trauma center. A *bebionic* myoelectric robotic hand and a motorized hook electric terminal device (ETD) (**Fig. 16**) are his preferred prosthetic devices for everyday use. The oilfield services company where he worked previously retasked him as a safety training specialist when he returned after his postinjury convalescence.

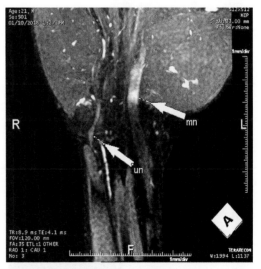

Fig. 11. MRN of partial hand amputation: un, ulnar nerve; mn, median nerve. Both the ulnar and median nerves had increased signal in the forearm, and the median nerve was flattened in the carpal tunnel with mild to moderate hyperintensity. No neuroma was seen in either nerve trunk.

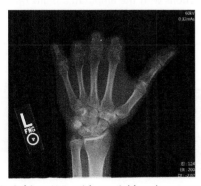

Fig. 10. Subject N.B. with partial hand amputation of the nondominant fingers at the proximal shaft of the proximal phalanges, posteroanterior (PA) radiograph.

EMG Summary Table										
	Spontaneous					MUAP				Recruitment
	IA	Fib	PSW	Fasc	H.F.	Amp	Dur.	PPP		Pattern
L. DELTOID	N	None	None	None	None	N	N	N		N
L. BICEPS	N	None	None	None	None	N	N	N		N
L. TRICEPS	N	None	None	None	None	N	N	N		N
L. PRON TERES	N	None	None	None	None	N	N	N		N
L. FIRST D INTEROSS	N	None	None	None	None	N	N	1+		N

Fig. 12. Preoperative EMG showed polyphasic action potentials in the first dorsal interosseous muscle, most likely because of local trauma at the time of his crush injury. IA, insertional activity; Fib, fibrillations; PSW, positive sharp waves; Fasc, fasciculations; H.F., high frequency; MUAP, motor unit action potentials; Dur., duration; Amp, amplitude; PPP, polyphasic potentials.

His dominant upper limb was amputated at midforearm level, in a position of fixed forearm pronation, which was typical for transradial amputees in our study (**Fig. 17**). MRN demonstrated diffuse thickening of the ulnar and median nerves throughout their course in the forearm, with terminal neuromas of both. There was minimal decrease in ulnar nerve and moderate decrease in median nerve diffusion tracts. Mild entrapment of the median nerve was seen at the exit of the nerve from the fibrous tunnel of the flexor digitorum superficialis (FDS) muscle origin, which is a

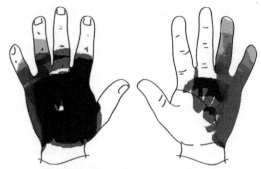

Fig. 14. Sensory stimulation of ulnar nerve sensory and motor fascicles, partial hand amputee. Ulnar sensory fascicle (*red*), ulnar motor fascicle (*blue*). Intensity of color indicates the frequency of receptive field activation during trials on different FAST-LIFE electrode channels.

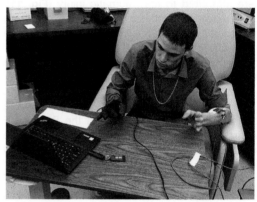

Fig. 15. Subject N.B. participating in motor signal recording and decoder training. "Ground truth" training data are collected from a motion tracking glove on the contralateral intact right hand, while neural signals are recorded from the FAST-LIFE electrodes in the amputated left upper limb. He performs real motions with the right hand while "imagining" hand motions with the amputated digits on the left hand.

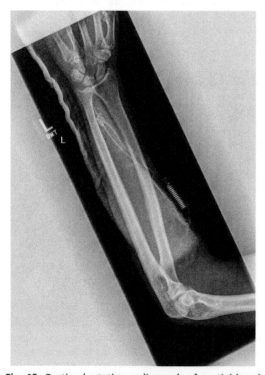

Fig. 13. Postimplantation radiograph of partial hand amputee, with FAST-LIFE electrodes implanted to the sensory and motor fascicles of the distal ulnar nerve.

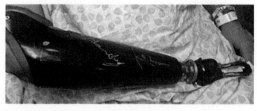

Fig. 16. Subject C.S. wearing his ETD robotic hook prosthesis, which he uses instead of his myoelectric robotic hand during heavy manual tasks.

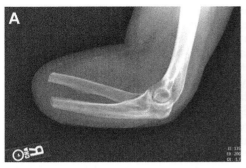
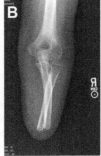

Fig. 17. Transradial amputation of the dominant upper limb at mid-forearm level: (*A*) radiograph, lateral view. (*B*) PA view.

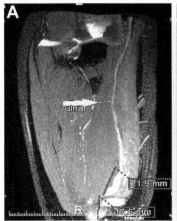
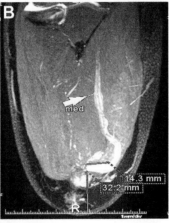

Fig. 18. MRN of transradial amputation stump: (*A*) ulnar nerve, (*B*) median nerve. Both nerves showed diffuse thickening and terminal neuromas. The median nerve was diagnosed with a site of anatomic compression at the fibrous origin of the FDS muscles.

EMG Summary Table									
	Spontaneous					MUAP			Recruitment
	IA	Fib	PSW	Fasc	H.F.	Amp	Dur.	PPP	Pattern
R. DELTOID	N	None	None	None	None	N	N	N	N
R. BICEPS	N	None	None	None	None	N	N	1+	N
R. TRICEPS	N	None	None	None	None	N	N	N	N
R. PRON TERES	N	None	None	None	None	N	N	N	N
R. FLEX CARPI ULN	N	None	None	None	None	N	N	2+	N
R. EXT CARPI R LONG	N	None	None	None	None	N	N	N	N
R. RHOMB MAJOR	N	None	None	None	None	N	N	1+	N

Fig. 19. Preoperative EMG showed intact function of median- and ulnar-innervated forearm muscles. IA, insertional activity; Fib, fibrillations; PSW, positive sharp waves; Fasc, fasciculations; H.F., high frequency; MUAP, motor unit action potentials; Dur., duration; Amp, amplitude; PPP, polyphasic potentials.

Impression:
1. This is an abnormal study.
2. There is electrodiagnostic evidence of right chronic C5 radiculopathy with signs of reinnervation and no signs of active denervation.

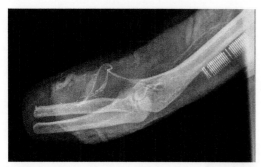

Fig. 20. Postimplantation radiograph of transradial amputee, with FAST-LIFE electrodes implanted to the sensory and motor fascicles of the median and ulnar nerves.

known site for proximal median nerve entrapment in pronator syndrome[6] (**Fig. 18**). EMG showed polyphasic action potentials in the nerves of the C5 distribution, indicating reinnervation with no signs of active denervation (**Fig. 19**).

Multichannel FAST-LIFE electrodes were implanted to the motor and sensory fascicular groups of the ulnar nerve, and to the thenar motor and thumb/index sensory fascicles of the median nerve. There were a total of 12 data channels per electrode, for a total of 48 channels. Wires from the FAST-LIFE electrodes were passed through the skin of the lateral arm and terminated in an external connector block (**Fig. 20**). When the median nerve was accessed for electrode implantation, we used a standard approach to the pronator tunnel where the dense, tight fascial band at the fibrous arch of FDS was identified and released.

Modified McGill pain questionnaire
(Postop values from POD#15)

Max pain	Preop	6.1
	Postop	2.8
Avg pain	Preop	2.1
	Postop	3.1
Descriptors	Preop	7
	Postop	7

Fig. 21. Modified McGill pain questionnaire results, from preoperative (preop) and postoperative (postop) day (POD) 15, reveal major improvement in pain following FAST-LIFE implantation surgery. Pain is graded on a Likert scale from 0 to 10. This most likely reflects decompression of his previously unrecognized pronator syndrome proximal median nerve compression, which began following his original traumatic injury.

Upon waking from surgery, the patient was noted to be inconsolably emotional in the recovery room. At his first postoperative clinic visit, he explained that the intractable neuropathic pain that he had experienced since the time of his initial injury was gone when he awoke from surgery. The modified McGill pain questionnaire that was collected during his clinic visits revealed major improvement (**Fig. 21**). These changes persisted throughout his participation in the study and continue to the time of this publication.

The patient was seen in our laboratory at UT Southwestern for experimental sessions weekly, beginning the week after implantation surgery. Motor recording to train the AI decoding algorithm was performed at the University of Minnesota. External connectors from the implanted FAST-LIFE electrodes were connected to a research electrophysiology system for sensory stimulation and motor recording (**Fig. 22**).

Sensory stimulation trials of the sensory and motor fascicles of the ulnar and median nerves were performed. These trials demonstrated expected findings of cutaneous sensation in the sensory fascicles and proprioceptive sensation in the motor fascicles, along the expected receptive fields based on the normal anatomic distribution of the nerves (**Fig. 23**).

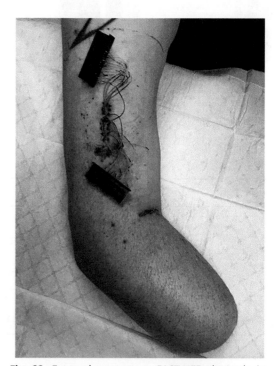

Fig. 22. External connectors, FAST-LIFE electrode interfaces in sensory and motor fascicles of median and ulnar nerves of transradial amputee.

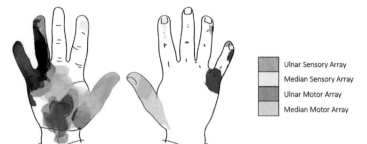

Ulnar Sensory Array
Median Sensory Array
Ulnar Motor Array
Median Motor Array

Fig. 23. Sensory stimulation of median and ulnar nerve sensory and motor fascicles, transradial amputee. Intensity of color indicates the frequency of receptive field activation during trials on different FAST-LIFE electrode channels.

As our scientific understanding and knowledge accumulated over the course of the study, our focus shifted increasingly to motor recording and decoding with later patients. With this patient, motor recording and decoding provided 15 DoF control of a robotic hand prosthesis. The patient's motor intent was decoded in real time and translated to control signals for a state-of-the-art robotic hand prosthesis (Video 3). Signal decodes were found to be durable over multiple weeks after initial training and provided the amputee with individual digit control of his prosthesis under a diverse set of experimental configurations (Video 4).

Explantation was performed uneventfully at 13 months after initial implantation. He has returned to normal use of his existing myoelectric robotic hand without any functional downgrade after his participation in the clinical trial.

SUMMARY

We have proven that the biology and physiology of the residual peripheral nerves of partial hand and transradial amputees are amenable to chronic FAST-LIFE electrode interfacing. By directing FAST-LIFE electrodes to the sensory- and motor-related intraneural components of the median and ulnar nerves, we can reliably restore tactile and proprioceptive sensation and record/decode motor signals informing high-fidelity robotic hand control. The ability to control a robotic hand prosthesis using intraneural electrode interfaces previously was thought to be technically impossible. In addition, these capabilities have been demonstrated in patients ranging from 9 months to 20 years after amputation, which provides reassurance that the native neural pathways for upper limb control remain viable and functional for decades after the limb has been missing.

FUTURE DIRECTIONS

The FAST-LIFE electrode interfacing approach has enabled us to perform chronic motor recording and intent decoding, with proprioceptive sensory restoration to provide feedback of voluntary motor activation. This approach has led us to the possibility of FAST-LIFE interfacing as a key to unlocking the basic physiology of motor control. In turn, FAST-LIFE interfacing holds promise as a tool to improve the understanding and treatment of motor control dysfunction resulting from several central and peripheral nervous system disorders, including stroke, spinal cord injury, brachial plexus injury, amyotrophic lateral sclerosis, Parkinson disease, and lower limb amputation.

CLINICS CARE POINTS

- Longitudinal intrafascicular electrodes can be individually targeted to the component fascicular groups within a peripheral nerve trunk without impairment of existing function.

- Expertise in intraneural anatomy and experience with meticulous microsurgical technique are required to handle the intraneural structures and place the implantable electrodes.

- Magnetic resonance neurography and electrodiagnostic studies can facilitate preoperative assessment of residual peripheral nerves within the amputation stump.

- Existing robotic hand prostheses using myoelectric control strategies are not capable of providing sensory feedback and reliable individual digit control of the robotic hand.

- It remains to be determined whether performing targeted muscle reinnervation surgery will eliminate options for future use of fascicle-specific targeting of longitudinal intrafascicular electrodes in the same patient for sensory feedback and peripheral nerve-derived motor control. We recommend counseling patients on this consideration regarding future technology before performing targeted muscle reinnervation surgery.

DISCLOSURE

J. Cheng and E. Keefer have ownership in Nerves Incorporated, which is a sponsor of the clinical studies described in this article using research funding provided by DARPA. Z. Yang is co-founder of, and holds equity in, Fasikl Inc, a sponsor of this project.

ACKNOWLEDGEMENT

We owe a great debt of gratitude to the wonderful patients who have given so generously of their time and their well-being by participating in this groundbreaking research. If there are heroes and angels to be found in this work, our patients deserve those accolades without any doubt. Our further efforts and our persistence in this work are now owed to them, as they have sacrificed for all amputees present and future, and we must succeed in bringing FAST-LIFE electrode interfacing to fruition as a standard-of-care clinical treatment in order to fully repay our debt to them.

SUPPLEMENTARY DATA

Supplementary data related to this article can be found online at https://doi.org/10.1016/j.hcl.2021.04.004.

REFERENCES

1. Perry BN, Moran CW, Armiger RS, et al. Initial clinical evaluation of the modular prosthetic limb. Front Neurol 2018;9:153.
2. Resnik L, Ekerholm S, Borgia M, et al. A national study of veterans with major upper limb amputation: survey methods, participants, and summary findings. PLoS One 2019;14(3). https://doi.org/10.1371/journal.pone.0213578.
3. Overstreet CK, Cheng J, Keefer EW. Fascicle specific targeting for selective peripheral nerve stimulation. J Neural Eng 2019;16(6). https://doi.org/10.1088/1741-2552/ab4370.
4. Oberlin C, Béal D, Leechavengvongs S, et al. Nerve transfer to biceps muscle using a part of ulnar nerve for C5-C6 avulsion of the brachial plexus: anatomical study and report of four cases. J Hand Surg Am 1994;19(2):232–7.
5. Tung TH, Novak CB, Mackinnon SE. Nerve transfers to the biceps and brachialis branches to improve elbow flexion strength after brachial plexus injuries. J Neurosurg 2003;98(2):313–8.
6. Cheng J, Mackinnon SE. Nerve transfers to restore pronation. In: Slutsky DJ, editor. Upper extremity nerve repair- tips and techniques: a master skills publication. Rosemont (IL): American Society for Surgery of the Hand; 2008. p. 213–26.
7. Cheng J, Mackinnon SE. Nerve transfers for digital sensation. In: Slutsky DJ, editor. Upper extremity nerve repair- tips and techniques: a master skills publication. Rosemont (IL): American Society for Surgery of the Hand; 2008. p. 181–92.
8. Lowe JB, Tung TR, Mackinnon SE. New surgical option for radial nerve paralysis. Plast Reconstr Surg 2002;110(3):836–43.
9. Hsiao EC, Fox IK, Tung TH, et al. Motor nerve transfers to restore extrinsic median nerve function: case report. Hand (N Y). 2009;4(1):92–7.
10. Kozin SH, Porter S, Clark P, et al. The contribution of the intrinsic muscles to grip and pinch strength. J Hand Surg Am 1999;24:64–72.
11. Nguyen AT, Xu J, Jiang M, et al. A bioelectric neural interface towards intuitive prosthetic control for amputees. J Neural Eng 2020. https://doi.org/10.1088/1741-2552/abc3d3.
12. Giladi A, Chung K. Surgical principles and perspectives on upper extremity amputations. In: Spires MC, Davis A, Kelly B, editors. Prosthetic restoration and rehabilitation of the upper and lower extremity. New York City: Demos Medical Publishing; 2013. p. 127–40.
13. Imbinto I, Peccia C, Controzzi M, et al. Treatment of the partial hand amputation: an engineering perspective. IEEE Rev Biomed Eng 2016;9:32–48.
14. Varma P, Stineman MG, Dillingham TR. Epidemiology of limb loss. Phys Med Rehabil Clin N Am 2014;25(1):1–8.
15. Singh Bhandari P, Deb P. Fascicular selection for nerve transfers: the role of the nerve stimulator when restoring elbow flexion in brachial plexus injuries. J Hand Surg 2011;36. https://doi.org/10.1016/j.jhsa.2011.08.017.
16. Kuiken TA, Barlow AK, Hargrove LJ, et al. Targeted muscle reinnervation for the upper and lower extremity. Tech Orthop 2017;32(2):109–16.
17. Wilbourn AJ. The electrodiagnostic examination with peripheral nerve injuries. Clin Plast Surg 2003;30:139–54.
18. Tam W-K, Wu T, Zhao Q, et al. Human motor decoding from neural signals: a review. BMC Biomed Eng 2019. https://doi.org/10.1186/s42490-019-0022-z.
19. Wu T, Zhao W, Keefer E, et al. Deep compressive autoencoder for action potential compression in large-scale neural recording. J Neural Eng 2018. https://doi.org/10.1088/1741-2552/aae18d.
20. Rincon-Gonzalez L, Warren JP, Meller DM, et al. Haptic interaction of touch and proprioception: implications for neuroprosthetics. IEEE Trans Neural Syst Rehabil Eng 2011;19(5):490–500.

Targeted Muscle Reinnervation for Prosthetic Control

Konstantin D. Bergmeister, MD, PhD[a,b,1], Stefan Salminger, MD, PhD[a,1], Oskar C. Aszmann, MD, PhD[a,*]

KEYWORDS

- TMR • Targeted muscle reinnervation • Prosthetics • Bionic reconstruction
- Reconstructive surgery

KEY POINTS

- Targeted muscle reinnervation (TMR) is the surgical rerouting of amputated nerves to remaining muscles of the stump.
- TMR increases the number of control signals for prosthetic control.
- TMR is most useful in transhumeral and glenohumeral amputees.
- Nerve transfers used in TMR change the neurophysiology of the motor unit.

TARGETED MUSCLE REINNERVATION
Nature of the Problem

Arm loss presents a significant lifetime event leading to severe physical and psychological burdens to patients. When limb salvage is futile, myoelectric prostheses can be used to restore limb function.[1,2] For the past 60 years, the amputee's agonist and antagonist muscle groups in the residual stump have been used as myocontrol signals for prosthetic control.[3–5] Although this control pattern is noninvasive, simple, and reliable, it is also limited to only 2 control signals from the agonist-antagonist muscle pair. In order to allow the control of more than 2 prosthetic functions, cocontraction (contracting agonist and antagonist muscles at the same time) is often used to switch prosthetic control of the different joints of the device (hand, wrist, elbow, or shoulder).[6,7] This traditional control method is not intuitive and cumbersome, but given its reliability is still the only widely used solution.[1,8] As modern myoelectric prostheses offer an increasing number of functions, this traditional control regime is insufficient to allow intuitive hand function.[2,9]

Development of Targeted Muscle Reinnervation

Targeted muscle reinnervation (TMR) was developed in the early 2000s in order to increase the number of intuitive control signals for prosthetic control.[10,11] In this procedure, amputated peripheral nerves in the affected extremity, which have lost their functional targets because of amputation, are surgically transferred to residual stump muscles after the original motor branch was divided. Thereby, the neuronal innervation of either segmentally innervated or multiheaded muscles (eg, biceps, pectoralis muscle) is surgically split, and thus, the number of available myosignals is increased.[12] Hereby, TMR enables the concurrent

---

[a] Clinical Laboratory for Bionic Extremity Reconstruction, Division of Plastic and Reconstructive Surgery, Department of Surgery, Medical University of Vienna, Vienna, Austria; [b] Department of Plastic, Reconstructive and Aesthetic Surgery, University Hospital St. Poelten, St. Poelten, Austria
[1] Contributed equally.
* Corresponding author.
E-mail address: oskar.aszmann@meduniwien.ac.at

Hand Clin 37 (2021) 415–424
https://doi.org/10.1016/j.hcl.2021.05.006

control of multiple prosthetic degrees of freedom (DoFs), such as wrist rotation, hand opening, and elbow flexion.[13] Following reinnervation of the target muscles, TMR control signals are easy and intuitive to use, as they have the same nerval innervation as the lost muscles that originally controlled that function. Therefore, the surgeon can make optimal use of the amputated nerve by surgically rerouting it to a new target muscle and simultaneously treating neuroma pain.[14] Thereby, patients may suffer less pain, which leads to better comfort while wearing the prosthesis and simultaneously have improved prosthetic function.

Indication

From a control perspective, transhumeral and glenohumeral amputees profit most from TMR surgery to improve prosthetic control. Generally, the more proximal the amputation is, the higher the need for robust control signals to replace the lost function and control the increased number of prosthetic joints. Patients with transradial or transcarpal amputation generally have a sufficient number of control signals to replace the missing hand. However, they may benefit from TMR for the therapy of neuroma or phantom limb pain.

Patients suitable for TMR surgery should have the necessary motivation and cognitive capacity to undergo time-consuming rehabilitation, which usually takes several months. Patients who are thought to be noncompliant are generally not suitable for TMR, given the extensive preoperative, intraoperative, and postoperative requirements. Likewise, patients should have a realistic expectation of the achievable prosthetic functionality, which is currently not comparable to a standard human hand.[15] Furthermore, as with every prosthetic fitting, patients will need lifelong support by a skilled prosthetist, and in the case of TMR, a Physical Medicine and Rehabilitation physician.

Preoperative Planning

From an anatomic perspective, the ideal TMR patient has sustained a sharp extremity amputation without significant soft tissue damage or brachial plexus injury.[11] This provides healthy nerves with sufficient length for the nerve transfers and healthy, intact residual innervated muscles. Possible neuromas of amputated nerves will be addressed during the surgery and do not pose a contraindication but may have an influence on the duration of the rehabilitation process. For patients with transhumeral amputations, the humerus should be 50% to 70% as long as it was before amputation. This is necessary to achieve sufficient prosthetic fitting and hence provide good functional outcome.[10,12] In addition, the remaining joints should have full range of motion. If not, prior physical therapy should be conducted to optimize total active and passive range of motion before TMR.

In cases that do not meet this prerequisite, additional procedures may have to be performed before TMR surgery. For example, patients with insufficient soft tissue coverage or lack of target muscles may need free flap transfer to reconstruct the absent tissue. Likewise, patients with a short humerus may require bone transfer or lengthening. These surgical modifications can be performed as a first step or addressed during TMR surgery, depending on the individual prerequisites of the residual limb.

Therefore, before surgery, the patient should be clinically evaluated to see if any of the above issues may be present so that a treatment plan can be developed. A thorough clinical examination of the brachial plexus is necessary to rule out any nerve injuries and determine whether the desired donor nerves and target muscles are present. For this purpose, neurophysiological analyses or imaging analyses may complete the presurgical examination. In the case of root avulsion, an MRI or MRI neurography can be used to evaluate whether there is any proximal root injury and to determine which nerves may be available for TMR. Conventional radiographs are often required to evaluate the skeletal properties of the residual limb.

Timing

If the affected arm has not had motor nerve damage, TMR can be done at virtually any time after the initial trauma. Some centers may even perform TMR during the initial trauma to prevent neuromas.[16] If a nerve or brachial plexus injury is present, the reconstruction should be done in a timely fashion to avoid the long-term consequences of muscle denervation, including muscle fibrosis and irreversible atrophy.

Preparation and Patient Positioning

The surgery is performed under general anesthesia, and no muscle relaxation should be administered because the donor motor nerves will need to be stimulated during surgery to evaluate the function of the nerves before nerve transfer. The patient is placed in a supine position with slight elevation of the shoulder for better access to the posterior shoulder and arm anatomic structures. The head is turned slightly to the opposite side, and the entire affected extremity, including the neck, is surgically prepared.

Procedural Approach

If there is a suspected injury to the brachial plexus, surgery begins with a supraclavicular exploration of the brachial plexus. This is particularly important if the brachial plexus has potentially suffered a traction injury, in order to both evaluate and treat possible proximal nerve damage. The subsequent steps depend on the level of amputation:

Transhumeral

1. In transhumeral amputees, the median, ulnar, and musculocutaneous nerves are accessed through a medial approach to the axillary fold.
2. Next, the motor branches of the musculocutaneous nerve innervating the brachial muscle and the medial and lateral heads of the biceps are identified and dissected free. This is essential to allow determination of the functionality of the different motor branches. Small-amplitude nerve stimulation (with a conventional nerve stimulator) should be sufficient to allow selective assessment of the targeted muscles.
3. Following identification of the target muscles and their respective motor branches, the short head of the biceps is dissected from the origin at the coracoid process and displaced to the medial distal aspect of the stump. This separates it distinctively from the long head of the biceps, especially for surface electromyographic (EMG) signal recording. Next, in above-elbow amputees, a subcutaneous fat flap is mobilized and placed between the short and the long head of the biceps to separate their EMG signals. Then, the subcutaneous fat above the targeted muscles is removed to maximize the signal amplitude when using surface EMG recording.
4. A lateral incision is then made, and the heads of the triceps are identified and dissected free. The lateral head is identified and isolated so that the motor branch can be dissected to its origin from the radial nerve. If the patient has a long stump and the proximal brachioradialis muscle is still intact, the distal radial nerve may be followed and split intraneurally into 2 components, which can be used to reinnervate the lateral head of the triceps and the brachioradialis muscle. Thereby, the overall number of muscles signals can be increased to allow separate hand opening and supination of the prosthesis.
5. Based on the anatomic prerequisites, the nerve transfer matrices described in **Fig. 1** are generally used in most transhumeral patients if possible.
6. If the standard transfer matrix is not possible due to nerve or muscle damage, the transfer must be adapted, and if required, the most necessary functions must be prioritized.
7. Amputated donor nerves are divided proximally to eliminate any neuromas present and to ensure that there are healthy nerve fascicles for the nerve transfer. The authors do not generally excise distal neuromas, as this would require additional, and often not beneficial, further dissection. The donor nerve is kept as long as possible to help achieve a tension-free nerve transfer.
8. Next, the motor branch to the target muscle is cut as distally as possible to minimize regeneration time. To prevent any aberrant

Amputation level	Targeted Muscles	Nerves	Prosthetic Function	Type of Innervation
	Biceps long head	Musculocutaneous	Elbow Flexion	Original
	Biceps short head	Ulnar	Hand Close	Transferred
	Brachialis	Median	Pronation	Transferred
Above elbow	Triceps long and medial head	Radial	Elbow Extension	Original
	Triceps lateral head	Split deep radial branch	Hand Open	Transferred
	Brachioradialis	Split deep radial branch	Supination	Transferred
	Pectoral major clavicular part	Musculocutaneous	Elbow Flexion	Transferred
	Pectoral minor	Ulnar	Hand Close	Transferred
Gleno-humeral	Pectoral major sternocostal part	Median	Hand Close/Wrist Rotation	Transferred
	Pectoral major abdominal part	Median	Wrist Rotation	Transferred
	Latissimus dorsi	Radial	Elbow Extension	Transferred
	Infraspinatus	Deep radial branch	Hand Open	Transferred

Fig. 1. TMR transfer matrix for transhumeral and glenohumeral amputees.

reinnervation, the proximal stump of the motor branch to the target muscle is resected proximally for a few centimeters and placed deep within tissue.

9. Then, the nerve transfers are performed microsurgically using loupe magnification with 8-0 or 9-0 monofilament sutures. The sutures should be tension free for optimal outcome, and the final repair should be secured additionally with fibrin glue.

10. If necessary, the shape of the residual limb can be improved by removing any excess soft tissue to facilitate prosthetic fitting.

Glenohumeral

1. The amputation scar on the thorax is reopened, and the pectoralis major muscle is exposed.

2. The pectoral nerves below the pectoral muscle are dissected from laterally to medially.

3. On the deep surface of the pectoralis muscles, the inferior, middle, and superior pectoral nerves to the clavicular, sternocostal, and abdominal portions of the pectoralis major muscle and the pectoralis minor muscle are identified and isolated.

4. With this level of amputation, the ulnar, median, musculocutaneous, and radial nerves are usually found in scar tissue. Therefore, meticulous neurolysis is required to identify the individual nerves based on their topography in relationship to the axillary artery. During this procedure, the thoracodorsal and suprascapular nerves to the latissimus dorsi and the infraspinatus muscle are identified as additional potential muscle signals.

5. To optimize the signal quality for surface EMG, the muscles are surgically separated to produce distinct myosignals. For this purpose, the origin of the pectoralis minor is dissected and mobilized, including its vascular supply to the midaxillary line.

6. For most patients, the nerve transfer matrix described in **Fig. 4** is suitable.

7. The target structures are explored, and all target muscles and donor nerves are tested to ensure that the desired functionality is achieved with the nerve transfers. If the standard transfer matrix is not possible because of nerve or muscle damage, the transfer must be adapted, and if required, the most necessary functions prioritized.

8. Amputated donor nerves are divided proximally to eliminate any neuromas present and to ensure that there are healthy nerve fascicles for the nerve transfer. Any additional length of

healthy nerve helps in achieving tension-free nerve transfers.

9. The motor branch to the target muscle is cut as distally as possible to minimize regeneration time. To prevent any aberrant reinnervation, the proximal stump of the motor branch to the target muscle is resected a few centimeters proximally and placed deep within tissue.

10. The nerve transfers are performed microsurgically using loupe magnification with monofilament 8-0 or 9-0 sutures. The sutures should be tension free for optimal outcome and secured using fibrin glue.

11. If necessary, the shape of the residual limb can be improved by removing any excess soft tissue to facilitate prosthetic fitting.

Management of Recovery and Rehabilitation

Following surgery and rehabilitation, the plasticity of the motor cortex allows the amputee to make use of the rewired neuromuscular structures and intuitively control the prosthesis in activities of daily living.[17,18] In transhumeral amputees, the long head of the biceps and the long and medial head of the triceps remain innervated; therefore, these prosthetic users may use their standard prosthesis throughout the postoperative rehabilitation process. Glenohumeral amputees will have to wait for sufficient reinnervation of the target muscles before prosthetic use. Within 3 to 9 months postoperatively, the reinnervation takes place, which is supported by a feedback-driven neurorehabilitation program to learn how to activate and separate the different signals. Here, EMG biofeedback is incorporated to facilitate motor learning and to help patients in learning how to activate the new muscle signals. This process is particularly difficult for patients who have sustained an amputation many years ago. In this case, a specifically trained rehabilitation program is necessary, under professional guidance of occupational therapists and physiotherapists to achieve optimal prosthetic rehabilitation. This is particularly relevant for the success of the surgery but unfortunately is often underestimated. For detailed information regarding this process, please refer to some of the previous published studies.[19–21] Regular outpatient visits are performed every few months to evaluate the progress of rehabilitation and determine if there are any short-term or long-term complications. Once the patient has become proficient with their prosthesis, the time intervals between clinical evaluations are increased.

Signal Acquisition

In conventional prosthesis without TMR, the few available muscle signals generally provide sufficient space to record EMG signals from surface electrodes individually. Following TMR, the high number of muscle signals in a relatively small area may be challenging for the prosthetist to enable individual recording of the signals. To address this issue, the novel muscle signals after TMR are spatially separated during the surgery to provide sufficient space between signals and thus facilitate recording with standard surface EMG electrodes.[12] Following rehabilitation, the TMR-EMG signals are usually independently controllable to provide separate prosthetic functions.

However, there are challenges with using surface EMG recordings, and it may require frequent visits to the prosthetist to optimize EMG recording sites or adapt the recoding sites to the changing shape of the residual limb. For example, the insufficient space between the individual muscles signals is challenging in transradial amputees. In glenohumeral amputees, the pectoralis major with its large surface may be challenging to record with standard EMG electrodes because of the size mismatch. Although surface EMG remains the gold standard with its reliability and easy-to-use application, novel technologies described in the future outlook section in later discussion promise additional signaling capacity.

Outcomes

TMR surgery is a safe procedure that has shown high success rates in multiple studies at centers with sufficient patient load.[13,22] Both function and comfort are improved in most patients undergoing TMR, which are the main factors for successful prosthetic use. Transhumeral amputees with sufficient stump length can generally achieve 6 individual and intuitive myosignals, using the described nerve transfers matrix, if the brachioradialis muscle is present. Thereby, it is possible to generate separate signals for each prosthetic DoF. In glenohumeral amputees, usually a maximum of 5 myoelectric signals is possible with the standard matrix.

For patients with either nerve damage or insufficient muscle signals or stump length, the most important goal is to achieve 4 individual muscle signals to enable the intuitive control of hand and elbow function. If possible, patients will benefit from 2 additional signals for wrist control. Consequently, in cases unsuitable for standard matrices, the surgeon should aim to perform nerve transfers of either the median or the ulnar nerve and one of the distal radial nerve branches.

If a patient has nerve damage that requires reconstruction, the nerve transfer matrix must focus on providing only cognitively "simple" nerve transfer, which facilitates rehabilitation. As an example, nerve transfers of median and ulnar nerves after repair may be difficult to cognitively separate during rehabilitation and subsequently for prosthetic use, as even in cases without nerve damage this is challenging.

Neurophysiology of Targeted Muscle Reinnervation

During TMR, the motor branch of a redundant muscle is cut and replaced by an amputated nerve. Thereby, the target muscle is reinnervated by another pool of motor neurons (**Figs. 2–4**). Thereby, the target muscle is linked and controlled by a new segment within the spinal cord and associated cortical areas, in comparison to its natural innervation. Following reinnervation and rehabilitation, TMR leads to reafferentation of the targeted muscle at the natural location of the missing limb within the homunculus.[23,24] This process of adaption of the cortex and spinal cord to the nerve transfers of TMR is the key feature that enables intuitive signals for prosthetic control. Here, the cortical areas originally linked to the fine motions of hand function are rerouted to proximal muscles of either the upper arm or the chest.

During this process, the nerve transfers used in TMR rewire the components of the motor units and change their physiology. Physiologically, the motor neuron with its axon and connected muscle fibers shares similar protein expression.[25,26] However, after a nerve transfer, motor neurons and their axons are linked to different muscle fibers, which may have different physiologic properties. Consequently, target muscle fibers change to the physiologic identity of the donor nerve and thus become physiologically similar to their original muscles.[27] Furthermore, most nerve transfers used in TMR are multifascicular nerves that usually innervate multiple nerves and instead are rerouted to single target muscles. This leads to hyper-reinnervation of the targeted muscle with smaller individually controllable motor units.[27–29] This surplus of potential axons for reinnervation and the short axonal regeneration distances for reinnervation are likely the reason for the high success rate of this procedure in terms of reinnervation.

Future Outlook of Targeted Muscle Reinnervation in Prosthetic Control

Although the above effects of TMR on the target muscle, such as muscle fiber adaption and hyper-reinnervation, are currently not used for

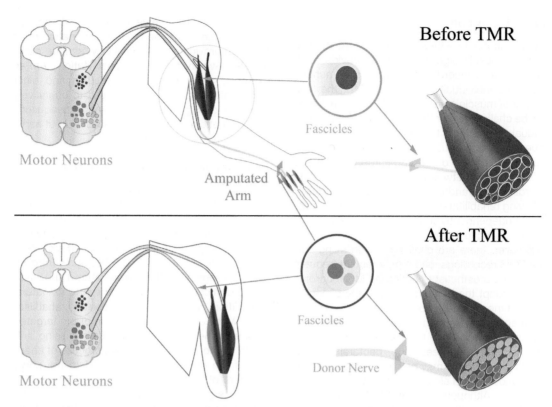

Fig. 2. Concept of TMR. (*top*) Before TMR, amputated nerves remain without function and may present with painful neuromas. (*bottom*) After TMR, the amputated nerve (in this case ulnar nerve) has been rerouted to the medial head of the biceps muscle in order to separate the innervation of the 2 heads. Consequently, 2 myosignals are available for prosthetic control. The donor nerve innervates the target muscle with its various fascicles and leads to changes in muscle fiber composition. (Picture from KD Bergmeister and colleagues[4] under Creative Commons Attribution License CC BY).

prosthetic control, experimental studies have shown their potential to further improve prosthetic control.[5,30–32] This additional control capacity is critical to control the latest experimental prosthetic devices, capable of highly dexterous and handlike motions with multiple DoFs and individual finger motions.[33–35] For controlling these many functions, a higher number of muscle signals than TMR currently provides are required.

In order to enable the recording of many more EMG signals, modern implantable EMG systems are promising, as they can acquire EMG signals in close proximity to other myosignals. Moreover, these implantable systems have been shown to provide stable relations between the muscle signal source and the implanted electrodes. This provides reliable signals even during motion, heavy loads on the prosthesis, and even if the patient is sweating. For example, epimysial or intramuscular implantation of EMG electrodes provides EMG signals that are not affected by the patient's subcutaneous tissues and do not change their location during repetitive use of the prosthesis.

These EMG systems are surgically implanted in the patient's extremity and record and wirelessly transmit high-quality muscle signals. Depending on the system's architecture, EMG information is recorded either epimysially from the muscle surface (eg, MyoPlant) or from within the muscle (eg, IMES). Thereby, even deep and/or small muscle signals can be easily recorded from muscle implants, resulting in an increase in control signals, which is not feasible with noninvasive EMG electrodes.

The MyoPlant system is one of the first of these systems and has successfully been tested in preclinical trials, where it showed good biocompatibility and reliable electrode impedance over many months. Furthermore, it was able to reliably record multiple adjacent EMG signals with distinct signal quality.[36–38] A different system developed by the Alfred Mann Foundation is the IMES system, that has already been clinically tested in patients with transradial amputations. Here, a set of 8 electrodes has been shown to be safe and has provided simple and efficient control over multiple DoFs in non-TMR patients.[39–41] Recently, a first

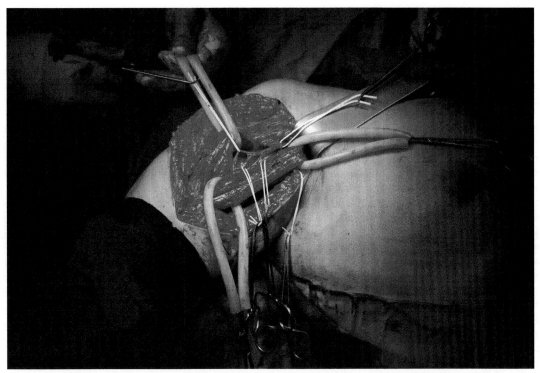

Fig. 3. Identification of the biceps and the musculocutaneous nerve before the nerve transfers.

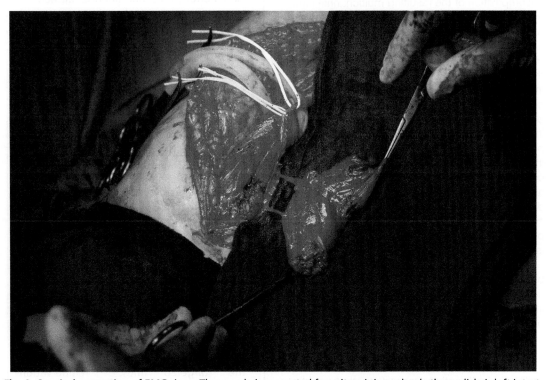

Fig. 4. Surgical separation of EMG signs. The muscle is separated from its origin and only the pedicle is left intact. Nerve transfers are performed to reinnervate the muscle as new EMG target signal.

patient trial has shown the improved prosthetic function after combined TMR surgery and IMES implantations in transhumeral amputees.[42]

In summary, implantable EMG electrodes are an exciting opportunity to further improve prosthetic control, especially in challenging locations, such as transhumeral and glenohumeral amputees.

Although prosthetic control is currently still far from natural hand motion, additional developments are being translated to the clinical arena to further increase the number of control signals. Based on recent advances in EMG decoding technology, it is now feasible to decode motor neuron activation from limited EMG data and thereby experimentally estimate the user's intended motion.[32,43] It has been shown that this approach is superior in TMR patients compared with classic pattern recognition in regard to less EMG interference in experimental settings.[32]

However, the required technology of high-density spatial sampling of EMG signals has only been recently implemented to intramuscular electrodes.[44,45] Hence, these systems are currently only suitable for acute experimental implantations but allow the identification of motor neurons in this setting.[45,46] Therefore, for the clinical translation of this development, the authors require multi-channel EMG electrodes that are safe for chronic implantation. Furthermore, online real-time decomposition of the resulting multichannel intramuscular signals is currently in development and has been shown only experimentally.[47]

A further development to improve prosthetic control is the use of osseointegration. Here, the prosthesis is connected to a socket that is implanted into the remaining bone of the residual limb.[48] This concept has been investigated in transhumeral amputees in combination with TMR and has shown increased range of motion, stable signals, and the possibility of sensory feedback as well.[49] The improved attachment to the body in comparison to conventional sockets provides more natural use and omits the problem of prosthesis displacement during heavy use. In addition, the direct skeletal connection provides the user with a sense of perception, termed osseoperception, where load is perceived via the bony attachment.

Hence, although much research is necessary before this exciting concept can be seen in patients, it is hoped it will provide a strong prosthetic interface for as many functions as the human hand or upper extremity can naturally perform.

SUMMARY

TMR has significantly advanced prosthetic control by increasing the number of control signals, making them more intuitive and treating neuromas at the same time. Patients with transhumeral or glenohumeral amputations benefit most from TMR from a control perspective, given the need for many reliable muscle signals. Correct patient selection for TMR surgery is vital, as patients require long and intensive rehabilitation. For many amputees, a standard nerve transfer matrix is feasible, which may be adapted to the individual patient. The success of the applied nerve transfers is high, which is in part due to transferring a surplus of axons to the target muscle and the short regeneration distance for the reinnervating nerve. With good adherence to rehabilitation and a well-designed prosthesis socket, patients can usually achieve a reliable improvement in prosthetic control. Neurophysiological insights into the mechanisms of TMR and novel implantable EMG systems are promising to further improve the control of prosthesis.

CLINICS CARE POINTS

- Evaluate if patient is a candidate for targeted muscle reinnervation by explaining the associated effort, time, and financial burden.

- Transhumeral and transradial amputees are most suitable for targeted muscle reinnervation to improve prosthetic control.

- Provide realistic information on what to expect from a targeted muscle reinnervation controlled prosthesis.

- Before surgery, the patient needs to be clinically examined for any nerve damage as a consequence of the amputation.

- Evaluate the shape of the residual limb and determine if any additional soft tissue is required, if the stump requires reshaping, or if the bone architecture is sufficient.

- Evaluate if standard nerve transfer matrices are suitable for the patient.

- Perform surgery beginning with treating any nerve damage, followed by the nerve transfers.

- Rehabilitation can be started after uneventful healing. Initial electromyographic signals are seen with biofeedback after typically 3 to 9 months.

- Prosthetic fitting should provide a stable interface and reliable signal acquisition of the targeted muscle reinnervation-electromyographic signals.

DISCLOSURE

The authors have nothing to disclose.

REFERENCES

1. Farina D, Aszmann O. Bionic limbs: clinical reality and academic promises. Sci Transl Med 2014; 6(257):257ps212.
2. Kung TA, Bueno RA, Alkhalefah GK, Langhals NB, Urbanchek MG, Cederna PS. Innovations in prosthetic interfaces for the upper extremity. Plast Reconstr Surg 2013;132(6):1515–23.
3. Childress DS. Historical aspects of powered limb prostheses. Clin Prosthet Orthot 1985;9(1):2–13.
4. Williams TW 3rd. Practical methods for controlling powered upper-extremity prostheses. Assist Technol 1990;2(1):3–18.
5. Parker P, Englehart K, Hudgins B. Myoelectric signal processing for control of powered limb prostheses. J Electromyogr Kinesiol 2006;16(6):541–8.
6. Aszmann OC, Roche AD, Salminger S, et al. Bionic reconstruction to restore hand function after brachial plexus injury: a case series of three patients. Lancet 2015;385(9983):2183–9.
7. Vujaklija I, Farina D, Aszmann O. New developments in prosthetic arm systems. Orthop Res Rev 2016;8: 31–9.
8. Turker KS. Electromyography: some methodological problems and issues. Phys Ther 1993;73(10): 698–710.
9. Ortiz-Catalan M, Branemark R, Hakansson B, Delbeke J. On the viability of implantable electrodes for the natural control of artificial limbs: review and discussion. Biomed Eng Online 2012;11:33.
10. Kuiken TA, Miller LA, Lipschutz RD, et al. Prosthetic command signals following targeted hyper-reinnervation nerve transfer surgery. Paper presented at: Annual International Conference of the IEEE Engineering in Medicine and Biology - Proceedings2005.
11. Miller LA, Stubblefield KA, Lipschutz RD, Lock BA, Kuiken TA. Improved myoelectric prosthesis control using targeted reinnervation surgery: a case series. IEEE Trans Neural Syst Rehabil Eng 2008;16(1): 46–50.
12. Dumanian GA, Ko JH, O'Shaughnessy KD, Kim PS, Wilson CJ, Kuiken TA. Targeted reinnervation for transhumeral amputees: current surgical technique and update on results. Plast Reconstr Surg 2009; 124(3):863–9.
13. Salminger S, Sturma A, Roche AD, Mayer JA, Gstoettner C, Aszmann OC. Outcomes, challenges, and pitfalls after targeted muscle reinnervation in high-level amputees: is it worth the effort? Plast Reconstr Surg 2019;144(6):1037e–43e.
14. Dumanian GA, Potter BK, Mioton LM, et al. Targeted muscle reinnervation treats neuroma and phantom pain in major limb amputees: a randomized clinical trial. Ann Surg 2019;270(2):238–46.
15. Bergmeister KD, Vujaklija I, Muceli S, et al. Broadband prosthetic interfaces: combining nerve transfers and implantable multichannel EMG technology to decode spinal motor neuron activity. Front Neurosci 2017;11:421.
16. Cheesborough JE, Souza JM, Dumanian GA, Bueno RA Jr. Targeted muscle reinnervation in the initial management of traumatic upper extremity amputation injury. Hand (N Y) 2014;9(2):253–7.
17. Stubblefield KA, Miller LA, Lipschutz RD, Kuiken TA. Occupational therapy protocol for amputees with targeted muscle reinnervation. J Rehabil Res Dev 2009;46(4):481–8.
18. Sturma A, Herceg M, Bischof B, Fialka-Moser V, Aszmann O. Rehabilitation following targeted muscle reinnervation in amputees. In: Jensen W, Andersen OK, Akay M, editors. Replace, repair, restore, relieve – bridging clinical and engineering solutions in neurorehabilitation, vol. 7. Springer International Publishing; 2014. p. 775–9.
19. Sturma A, Hruby LA, Farina D, Aszmann OC. Structured motor rehabilitation after selective nerve transfers. J Vis Exp 2019;(150).
20. Sturma A, Hruby LA, Prahm C, Mayer JA, Aszmann OC. Rehabilitation of upper extremity nerve injuries using surface EMG biofeedback: protocols for clinical application. Front Neurosci 2018;12:906.
21. Sturma A, Roche AD, Göbel P, et al. A surface EMG test tool to measure proportional prosthetic control. Biomed Tech (Berl) 2015;60(3):207–13.
22. Kuiken TA, Li G, Lock BA, et al. Targeted muscle reinnervation for real-time myoelectric control of multifunction artificial arms. JAMA 2009;301(6):619–28.
23. Yao J, Chen A, Kuiken T, Carmona C, Dewald J. Sensory cortical re-mapping following upper-limb amputation and subsequent targeted reinnervation: a case report. Neuroimage Clin 2015;8:329–36.
24. Chen A, Yao J, Kuiken T, Dewald JP. Cortical motor activity and reorganization following upper-limb amputation and subsequent targeted reinnervation. Neuroimage Clin 2013;3:498–506.
25. Heckman CJ, Enoka RM. Motor unit. Compr Physiol 2012;2(4):2629–82.
26. Buchthal F, Schmalbruch H. Motor unit of mammalian muscle. Physiol Rev 1980;60(1):90–142.
27. Bergmeister KD, Aman M, Muceli S, et al. Peripheral nerve transfers change target muscle structure and function. Sci Adv 2019;5(1):eaau2956.
28. Kuiken TA, Childress DS, Rymer WZ. The hyper-reinnervation of rat skeletal muscle. Brain Res 1995 Apr 3;676(1):113–23. https://doi.org/10.1016/0006-8993 (95)00102-v. PMID: 7796162.
29. Kapelner T, Jiang N, Holobar A, et al. Motor unit characteristics after targeted muscle reinnervation. PLoS One 2016;11(2):e0149772.

30. Farina D, Merletti R, Enoka RM. The extraction of neural strategies from the surface EMG: an update. J Appl Physiol (1985) 2014;117(11):1215–30.

31. Muceli S, Bergmeister KD, Hoffmann KP, et al. Decoding motor neuron activity from epimysial thin-film electrode recordings following targeted muscle reinnervation. J Neural Eng 2019;16(1):016010.

32. Farina D, Vujaklija I, Sartori M, et al. Man/machine interface based on the discharge timings of spinal motor neurons after targeted muscle reinnervation. Nat Biomed Eng 2017;1:0025.

33. Resnik L, Klinger SL, Etter K. The DEKA arm: its features, functionality, and evolution during the Veterans Affairs Study to optimize the DEKA Arm. Prosthet Orthot Int 2014;38(6):492–504.

34. Fifer MS, Hotson G, Wester BA, et al. Simultaneous neural control of simple reaching and grasping with the modular prosthetic limb using intracranial EEG. IEEE Trans Neural Syst Rehabil Eng 2014; 22(3):695–705.

35. Lee B, Attenello FJ, Liu CY, McLoughlin MP, Apuzzo ML. Recapitulating flesh with silicon and steel: advancements in upper extremity robotic prosthetics. World Neurosurg 2014;81(5-6):730–41.

36. Poppendieck W, Ruff R, Gail A, et al. Evaluation of implantable epimysial electrodes as possible interface to control myoelectric hand prostheses 2011.

37. Lewis S, Hahn M, Klein C, et al. Implantable silicone electrode for measurement of muscle activity: results of first in vivo evaluation. Biomed Tech (Berl) 2013.

38. Bergmeister KD, Hader M, Lewis S, et al. Prosthesis control with an implantable multichannel wireless electromyography system for high-level amputees: a large-animal study. Plast Reconstr Surg 2016; 137(1):153–62.

39. Pasquina PF, Evangelista M, Carvalho AJ, et al. First-in-man demonstration of a fully implanted myoelectric sensors system to control an advanced electromechanical prosthetic hand. J Neurosci Methods 2014.

40. Baker JJ, Scheme E, Englehart K, Hutchinson DT, Greger B. Continuous detection and decoding of dexterous finger flexions with implantable myoelectric sensors. IEEE Trans Neural Syst Rehabil Eng 2010;18(4):424–32.

41. Weir RF, Troyk PR, DeMichele G, et al. Implantable myoelectric sensors (IMES) for upper-extremity prosthesis control- preliminary work. Paper presented at: Engineering in Medicine and Biology Society, 2003. Proceedings of the 25th Annual International Conference of the IEEE; 17-21 September 2003, 2003.

42. Salminger S, Sturma A, Hofer C, et al. Long-term implant of intramuscular sensors and nerve transfers for wireless control of robotic arms in above-elbow amputees. Sci Robot 2019;4(32):eaaw6306.

43. Kapelner T, Ning J, Vujaklija I, et al. Classification of motor unit activity following targeted muscle reinnervation. Paper presented at: Neural Engineering (NER), 2015 7th International IEEE/EMBS Conference on; 22-24 April 2015, 2015.

44. Farina D, Yoshida K, Stieglitz T, Koch KP. Multi-channel thin-film electrode for intramuscular electromyographic recordings. J Appl Physiol (1985) 2008; 104(3):821–7.

45. Muceli S, Poppendieck W, Negro F, et al. Accurate and representative decoding of the neural drive to muscles in humans with multi-channel intramuscular thin-film electrodes. J Physiol 2015;593(17): 3789–804.

46. Negro F, Muceli S, Castronovo AM, Holobar A, Farina D. Multi-channel intramuscular and surface EMG decomposition by convolutive blind source separation. J Neural Eng 2016;13(2):026027.

47. Karimimehr S, Marateb HR, Muceli S, Mansourian M, Mananas MA, Farina D. A real-time method for decoding the neural drive to muscles using single-channel intra-muscular EMG recordings. Int J Neural Syst 2017;1750025.

48. Aman M, Festin C, Sporer ME, et al. Bionic reconstruction : restoration of extremity function with osseointegrated and mind-controlled prostheses. Wien Klin Wochenschr 2019;131(23-24):599–607.

49. Ortiz-Catalan M, Mastinu E, Sassu P, Aszmann O, Brånemark R. Self-contained neuromusculoskeletal arm prostheses. N Engl J Med 2020;382(18): 1732–8.

Regenerative Peripheral Nerve Interfaces for Advanced Control of Upper Extremity Prosthetic Devices

Nishant Ganesh Kumar, MD[a], Theodore A. Kung, MD[a], Paul S. Cederna, MD[b,c],*

KEYWORDS

- Amputation • Neuroprosthetic control • Regenerative peripheral nerve interface • RPNI
- Prosthetic control

KEY POINTS

- Although prosthetic device technology has rapidly evolved over the past few decades, current prosthetic limbs are unable to replicate the complex functions of the upper extremity because of the lack of an ideal interface between the prosthesis and residual limb. An ideal neuroprosthetic interface should transduce volitional motor control signals with high signal-to-noise ratios, require minimal recalibration, demonstrate long-term durability and signal stability, and be safe to use.
- Broadly classified, current prosthetic device control strategies involve myoelectric control using residual muscles within the remaining limb, brain computer interfaces to record motor signals from the brain, and peripheral nerve interfaces that use electrodes to harness signals directly from peripheral nerves in the residual limb. Unfortunately, these techniques are limited in their ability to sustain long-term prosthesis control with high reliability and specificity.
- The regenerative peripheral nerve interface (RPNI) comprises a free autologous skeletal muscle graft that can be secured around the terminal end of a peripheral nerve or individual fascicles in a residual limb. Animal studies have demonstrated durability, stability, and reliability of RPNIs in transducing peripheral nerve signals with high signal-to-noise ratios to execute volitional and continuous finger movements in a prosthetic hand.
- By acting as an amplifier of efferent motor signals, RPNIs have been used successfully in humans to control an artificial hand with high specificity without the need for constant control algorithm recalibration. Given its promising clinical results, RPNIs have the potential to revolutionize prosthetic device control for patients living with amputation.

 Video content accompanies this article at http://www.hand.theclinics.com.

INTRODUCTION

For decades, the most popular type of prosthetic device was a body-powered prosthesis that used a series of cables, harnesses, and rubber bands to control a prosthesis. Although body-powered prosthetic devices still are used today and can

---

[a] Section of Plastic Surgery, Department of Surgery, University of Michigan, 2130 Taubman Center, 1500 East Medical Center Drive, Ann Arbor, MI 48109-0340, USA; [b] Section of Plastic Surgery, Department of Surgery, University of Michigan, 2130 Taubman Center, 1500 East Medical Center Drive, Ann Arbor, MI 48109-0340, USA; [c] Department of Biomedical Engineering, University of Michigan, Ann Arbor, MI, USA
* Corresponding author. Section of Plastic Surgery, Department of Surgery, University of Michigan, 2130 Taubman Center, 1500 East Medical Center Drive, Ann Arbor, MI 48109-0340.
E-mail address: cederna@med.umich.edu

Hand Clin 37 (2021) 425–433
https://doi.org/10.1016/j.hcl.2021.04.005

meet the functional needs of many individuals with amputation, such devices lack intuitive control.[1,2] The desire to develop an intuitive prosthetic device control strategy that enables volitional, real-time, and coordinated movements has spurred the development of novel interfaces between the prosthetic device and its user.

The most recent surgical technique to demonstrate enhanced prosthetic device control capabilities is the regenerative peripheral nerve interface (RPNI). The RPNI comprises an autologous free skeletal muscle graft secured around the terminal end of a peripheral nerve or individual fascicles of a peripheral nerve (**Fig. 1**).[3] Since its initial development and subsequent validation in successfully transducing peripheral nerve signals for reliable and specific upper extremity prosthetic device control, RPNIs have been used in humans to control an artificial hand. This article reviews the current strategies for neuroprosthetic control, its limitations, and the subsequent development and use of RPNIs for intuitive and advanced prosthetic device control.

CURRENT PROSTHETIC DEVICE CONTROL STRATEGIES

Early prosthetic device fitting and initiation of rehabilitation are advocated to achieve optimal functional restoration in patients with upper extremity amputations.[4] This is important particularly in this patient population who typically are young and healthy and have many years of productive employment ahead of them.[5] Successfully encouraging prosthetic device use and rehabilitation among upper limb amputation patients depends on having a prosthetic device that is functional and easy to use. Evidence suggests that the use of myoelectric prosthetic devices that offer more functionality are associated with increased use regardless of amputation level compared with passive prosthetic devices.[5] In the recent past, several advancements have been made in developing functional prosthetic devices. Unfortunately, despite advances in prosthetic device technology, device fabrication, engineered materials, and signal processing methods, the true potential of prosthetic devices is yet to be achieved due to a lack of integrated and intuitive control.[6–8] This need to develop a reliable interface between the residual limb and prosthesis to facilitate intuitive neuroprosthetic control has resulted in the ongoing evolution of 3 major types of control strategies, which involve interfacing with: (1) residual muscle groups (myoelectric control); (2) the central nervous system (brain-computer interfaces [BCIs]); and (3) the peripheral nervous system (peripheral nerve interfaces [PNIs]).[9]

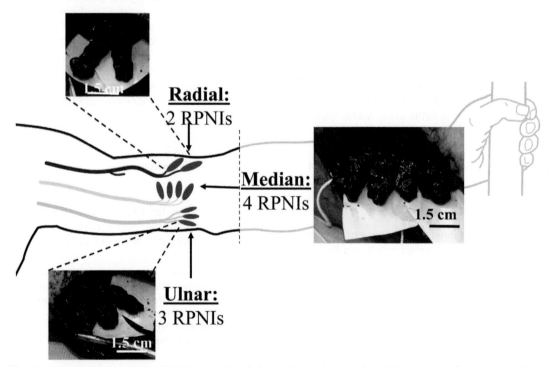

Fig. 1. Intraoperative creation of RPNI. Fascicles of the median, ulnar, and radial nerves are dissected out. Creation of RPNIs surrounding the fascicles of these major peripheral nerves is performed using free autologous skeletal muscle grafts.

Myoelectric prosthetic control uses surface electrodes to detect electromyogram (EMG) signals from residual muscles and currently is the most common method of neuroprosthetic control.[9] Several myoelectric systems can be used with commercially available prosthetic devices, which has led to widespread adoption. EMG signals can be recorded using both invasive and noninvasive techniques. Noninvasive EMG recording techniques are preferred because invasive EMG recording techniques, although more specific, are too burdensome for users.[10] Surface EMGs can be recorded using dry electrodes or wet electrodes. In general, dry electrodes are preferred to wet electrodes because of the difficulties in attaching wet electrodes securely and the high costs associated with these systems.[10] Unfortunately, the use of dry electrodes for surface EMG control is suboptimal due to high electrical impedance between the skin and electrode from motion, body hair, and sweat. In addition, myoelectric systems are less useful for prosthetic device control because they require frequent control-algorithm calibrations, have decreased signal-to-noise ratios (SNRs), and lack intuitive motor control.[6,9,10]

For many years, scientists and engineers have been developing approaches to control prosthetic devices by recording volitional motor signals directly from the brain.[11] BCIs or brain-machine interfaces can record electrical activity from the scalp, from the surface of the brain, or from within the motor cortex of the brain.[11] BCIs are useful interface strategies in patients without functional peripheral nerves or in patients with spinal cord injury that preclude the use of peripheral nerves as a source of signals for prosthesis control. BCIs also recently have been used in neurorehabilitation in paraplegic patients.[12–15]

Signals in BCIs can be recorded via 4 primary methods: (1) electroencephalography (EEG); (2) electrocorticography (ECoG); (3) local field potentials; and (4) single-neuron action potential recordings.[11] EEG, although noninvasive because it records signals from the surface of the scalp, has poorer spatial resolution in signal recording. The distance of 2 cm to 3 cm from the electrode tips to the cortex of the brain negatively affects the quality of the signals being recorded.[11] Other techniques, such as ECoG and the use of electrodes directly on the surface of the brain or within the brain cortex, are fraught with risk due to the need of an invasive operation. Furthermore, the inability to guarantee stable performance and signal recording over a period of time, migration and motion of electrodes, neuronal injury during insertion, device encapsulation, and acute and chronic inflammation affect the reliability of signals captured using invasive cortical recording techniques.[11,16] Nevertheless, ECoG has demonstrated the potential for real-time control of a prosthetic hand in a poststroke patient and in the control of a prosthetic arm in patients with paralysis but without sensorimotor cortex injury.[17,18] As the operative and long-term safety of such procedures is established, invasive BCIs represent a viable neuroprosthetic option for select patients without peripheral nerve targets.

PNIs have been designed to record signals directly from peripheral nerves. Electrode interfaces in the peripheral nervous system can be classified broadly as extraneural, intraneural, and regenerative.[19] Extraneural PNIs, such as cuff electrodes, offer lower signal capturing selectivity compared with intraneural PNIs because they are wrapped around the nerve externally. In contrast, intraneural PNIs, such as penetrating arrays, offer greater selectivity at the cost of potential neural injury, inflammation, and encapsulation from device implantation.[20] Regenerative electrodes (such as the sieve electrode) were designed as sieves or hollow electrode arrays between severed nerves such that the nerve grows through an array of holes and electrodes around each hole interface with the sprouting axon.[9,19] Although this was meant to improve selectivity, its use has been demonstrated mainly in animal models with mixed results because some studies have shown evidence of axonal damage from compression, motion at the biotic-abiotic interface, and challenging signal recording due to disorganized nerve growth.[19,21]

Given the limitations of these interfacing strategies, there was a need to design a prosthetic device interface that maximizes signal recordings with high SNRs and enables signal specificity to execute the functions of an upper extremity. In addition, such an interface needed to minimize damage to the delicate neural microenvironment from inflammation and biofouling, which occurs with invasive signal-recording interfaces. Furthermore, such an interface needed to be durable and stable over a long-period of time to facilitate reliable long-term prosthetic device control. Lastly, the interface needed to decrease neuroma formation, which could lead to significant user pain, hinder prosthetic use, create signal interference from aberrant axonal sprouting, and affect signal quality by inappropriately low depolarization potentials.[22]

Skeletal muscle has been recognized as an attractive option for neuroprosthetic interfacing because of its regenerative potential and the greater amplitude of EMG signals generated from contracting muscle compared with neural signals, making these volitional motor signals easier to record.[9,23] The RPNI takes advantage of this property of skeletal muscle to overcome the disadvantages of existing prosthetic device control strategies. It comprises a free autologous skeletal muscle graft secured around the terminal end of a peripheral nerve or individual fascicles.

After the free skeletal muscle graft is secured around the terminal end of the nerve or fascicle, the muscle graft undergoes a process of degeneration, regeneration, and reinnervation.[24] As with any free tissue graft (eg, skin graft), the skeletal muscle graft initially is supported by imbibition, after which it undergoes inosculation and revascularization.[25,26] During the regenerating process, the acutely denervated muscle graft undergoes reinnervation by the secured peripheral nerve or fascicle to create new neuromuscular junctions. An electrode then is implanted in the RPNI to record specific efferent motor action potentials.[24] By having electrodes interface with a muscle, RPNIs avoid the iatrogenic axonal injury that occurs when electrodes directly interface with peripheral nerves. Furthermore, the RPNI decreases neuroma formation and aberrant axonal regeneration that affect signal quality and amplifies efferent motor action potentials, which improves SNRs in recorded signals.[27] Because individual fascicles can be used to create RPNIs, selective and specific prosthetic device control to support multiple degrees of freedom is possible. This leads to a more enhanced and intuitive experience compared with current neuroprosthetic control strategies.

DEVELOPMENT OF THE REGENERATIVE PERIPHERAL NERVE INTERFACE
Successful Recording of Compound Muscle Action Potentials from Regenerative Peripheral Nerve Interfaces

Prior to its use in humans, extensive preliminary testing of RPNIs was conducted using animal models. Initial testing that utilized divided peroneal nerves in rats showed that RPNIs were reinnervated and revascularized successfully, with histologic evidence of axonal regeneration and synaptogenesis within the RPNI.[22] With reinnervation, relatively low-amplitude efferent motor action potentials created high-amplitude compound muscle action potentials (CMAPs) in the RPNI that easily were recorded.[22] This demonstrated the ability of RPNIs to serve as a bioamplifier of peripheral nerve signals.

Subsequent experiments in rats revealed that RPNIs enabled stable and reliable signal transduction in real-time during voluntary muscle activation

to enable control of a prosthetic hand.[28] RPNIs had higher SNRs compared with a control group without RPNIs. In addition, these studies found that RPNI EMG activity was not significantly affected by motion artifact or cross-talk from neighboring muscles.[28] Therefore, these studies helped establish the ability of RPNIs to facilitate real-time neuroprosthetic control with high SNRs and minimal signal contamination from adjacent muscles.

To demonstrate long-term stability of RPNIs and their ability to transduce efferent motor action potentials into CMAPs, a rat hind limb amputation model has been used.[29,30] RPNIs were created on the end of the transected peroneal nerve. Signal recordings then were measured at 12-months and 14-months postoperatively and demonstrated large-amplitude CMAPs with no evidence of RPNI degeneration or signal degradation with time. At 14 months, RPNIs were viable, reinnervated, and capable of signal generation.[30] Importantly, despite repeated stimulation, large-amplitude signals consistently were transduced using RPNIs. These studies demonstrated that RPNIs were a stable and reliable PNI that facilitated transduction of efferent motor action potentials into large-amplitude CMAPs, with favorable SNRs, over long time-periods.

After demonstrating the safety of RPNIs in rodent models, RPNIs subsequently were evaluated in rhesus macaques. In these experiments, RPNIs were created using the median and radial nerves, and the monkeys were trained to perform a finger movement task that required simultaneous movements of 4 fingers.[31] EMG signals recorded from the RPNIs for finger flexion, finger rest, and finger extension had an accuracy greater than 96%. Long-term stability in this nonhuman primate model was demonstrated with efferent motor action potentials transduced to large-amplitude CMAPs with high SNRs for up to 20 months postimplantation.[31] These experiments were important to demonstrate that the RPNIs were safe and caused no functional deficits in the monkeys.[31] The RPNIs produced normal and volitional EMG signals of high quality to enable functional prosthetic device control to execute discrete finger movement tasks with high accuracy. This work was advanced in subsequent testing on rhesus macaques to control continuous and real-time finger flexion and extension of a prosthetic hand using indwelling electrodes.[32] Together, these animal studies laid the ground work for clinical testing of RPNIs in humans with upper extremity amputations.

USE OF REGENERATIVE PERIPHERAL NERVE INTERFACE IN HUMANS FOR PROSTHETIC DEVICE CONTROL

To optimize functional restoration following limb loss, RPNIs should be created on all nerves and nerve fascicles responsible for upper limb and hand function. If feasible, fascicular RPNIs should be created on all major peripheral nerves to enable more high-fidelity prosthetic control with greater degrees of freedom. For instance, in 1 patient with a prior proximal transradial amputation, 4 RPNIs were created on the median nerve, 3 on the ulnar nerve, and 2 for the radial nerve (see **Fig. 1**).[33] Donor skeletal muscle can be harvested from the site of amputation (eg, brachioradialis in the upper extremity) or distant from the site of amputation (eg, vastus lateralis in the lower extremity).

RPNIs have been used successfully in humans for real-time prosthetic device control in patients with an upper extremity amputation.[33] In the pilot study, the levels of amputation in the patients included were transradial, glenohumeral, and wrist disarticulation. In these patients, RPNIs were created by first dissecting out the distal ends of transected residual nerves that included the median nerve, ulnar nerve, and radial nerve. Next, autologous free skeletal muscle grafts measuring approximately 3.0 cm × 2.0 cm × 0.5 cm were obtained from the patient's native vastus lateralis. These skeletal muscle grafts were then secured around the terminal end of a residual peripheral nerve fascicle to create individual fascicular RPNIs. In this pilot study, signals were recorded using surface EMG or percutaneous wires from the RPNIs or with surgically implanted indwelling bipolar electrodes.

In humans, RPNIs were shown to transduce efferent motor action potentials into large-amplitude CMAPs with high SNRs for high-fidelity prosthetic control of both extrinsic and intrinsic hand and finger functions.[33] Compared with other methods of harnessing signals directly from nerves, including cuff and intraneural electrodes, patients who underwent implantation of indwelling bipolar EMG electrodes into their RPNIs had higher SNRs for prosthetic control. Specifically, the highest mean SNR in human trials was 68.9, which is substantially higher compared with measured SNRs in nerve cuff electrodes and intraneural probes that range from 4 to 15. Even in patients where surface and epimysial EMG signals were recorded from innervated residual muscles of the limb, the SNR still ranged only from 9 to 35.[33–38] Furthermore, unlike electrodes that directly interface with the nerve causing iatrogenic neural injury and issues with signal stability and degradation, RPNIs did not create neural damage and remained stable in patients for up to 3 years with unchanged signal amplitude.[33]

Through ultrasound imaging, human trials also showed the functional selectivity of RPNIs. For instance, in 1 of the patients with multiple median nerve RPNIs, independent contractions of the RPNIs during thumb interphalangeal joint flexion, index finger proximal interphalangeal (PIP) joint, and index finger distal interphalangeal (DIP) joint flexion were observed independently. Subsections of the same RPNI and alternative RPNIs of the median nerve fascicles were shown to contract on ultrasound based on different motor intent. This indicates that a given RPNI has individual motor units that contract independent of each other, which permits recording signals with high specificity. To enable selective and functional prosthetic control, electrodes can be spaced out millimeters apart on the large surface area of the skeletal muscle graft in an RPNI, to record signals with high specificity. This overcomes a significant barrier to PNIs that require micrometer spacing of intraneural electrodes to record specific signals from peripheral nerves.[33]

In addition to the median nerve, RPNIs also were created successfully with the ulnar nerve. These RPNIs were shown on ultrasound to contract during voluntary flexion of the small finger PIP and DIP. In addition, ulnar RPNIs were involved in thumb movement consistent with anatomic innervation of intrinsic musculature of the thumb. Of great promise, in a patient with a shoulder-level amputation, distinct RPNIs were identified that facilitated individual finger movement. This highlights a key advantage of RPNIs over other techniques. Because it harnesses signals directly from peripheral nerves, RPNIs do not rely on intrinsic or extrinsic musculature. Instead, fascicular RPNIs can be used to capture signals responsible for intrinsic finger movement even in patients with proximal amputations in the upper extremity.

Similar to results in animal experiments, patients were able to voluntarily control RPNI signals for continuous control of prosthetic finger movements with high accuracy over a long period of time (Video 1).[33] In experimental tasks to demonstrate the accuracy of prosthetic control, patients completed tasks with high accuracy (96%–100%) on day 0 and up to day 300 (96%–100%). Furthermore, signal amplitudes were maintained during such recordings. Patients had the ability to control multiple degrees of freedom of the thumb with high accuracy during performance tasks. These included movement of the thumb at the IP joint and the thumb carpometacarpal and metacarpophalangeal joints. From a patient perspective, prosthetic device control was feasible using RPNI signals without the need for control algorithm recalibration. This is a significant advance in prosthetic device control because existing strategies require frequent calibrations for reliable control. Together, these findings establish the high reliability, stability, and durability of RPNIs in peripheral nerve signal transduction for enhanced and intuitive prosthetic device control.

In discussing the use of RPNIs for neuroprosthetic control, it is worth highlighting targeted muscle reinnervation (TMR). Briefly, TMR involves a nerve transfer procedure wherein residual peripheral nerves in an amputated limb are transferred to a motor nerve branch of a target muscle.[39] After reinnervation by the residual peripheral nerve, contraction of the target muscle can be recorded by surface EMG to facilitate prosthetic device control. TMR has been performed successfully in patients with shoulder, transhumeral, and transradial amputations to facilitate prosthetic control of the upper extremity involving the elbow, hand, and fingers.[39–41] Compared with conventional myoelectric control, TMR enables simultaneous control of discrete functions in different regions of the upper extremity, such as elbow and hand, instead of traditional mode switching methods that were used prior to TMR.[41] Furthermore, similar to the use of pattern recognition control of an artificial hand using RPNIs,[33] TMR has been shown to implement pattern recognition control of prosthetic devices successfully in patients with transhumeral amputations.[42] Using pattern recognition control of prosthetic devices, TMR patients performed statistically better on tasks that required movements along 3 degrees of freedom than patients using direct control of prosthetic devices.[42]

A key difference between TMR and RPNI is that TMR requires partial denervation of a target muscle for reinnervation by a residual peripheral nerve. For high-level amputations (eg, shoulder disarticulation) the same target muscle (eg, sternal head of pectoralis) may be used for multiple residual nerves (eg, median and ulnar nerve).[41] Because the peripheral nerve signals are recorded using surface EMG, signal specificity is diminished compared with RPNIs, where signals are recorded on a fascicular level. From a prosthetic control standpoint, this could limit the number of independent movements using TMR compared with RPNIs, because fascicular RPNIs have the potential for a higher number of degrees of freedom of prosthesis control.[33] Furthermore, prosthetic system designs need to be tailored for each patient in TMR and require more frequent calibrations

compared with RPNIs.[33,43] Lastly, because it currently is reliant on surface EMG to record signals, TMR suffers from similar issues affecting surface myoelectric systems, such as signal interference at the skin-electrode interface.[9] The success of indwelling electrodes in patients with RPNIs, and its long-term stability in high-quality signal transduction, means that combined with wireless signal recording technology, RPNIs can bypass the limitations of surface recording systems.[33] Such wireless systems currently are being developed for use in humans.

Despite these differences, it is possible that the ideal motor control interface for prosthetic devices involves a combination of TMR and RPNI techniques that leverages the benefits of TMR and the ability of RPNIs to enable multiple independent control sites. TMR has provided a significant advance in the functional restoration of patients following limb loss and will undoubtedly play an important role into the future.

FUTURE DIRECTIONS AND APPLICATIONS OF REGENERATIVE PERIPHERAL NERVE INTERFACES IN ENHANCING PROSTHETIC EXPERIENCE

Integrating sensory feedback to create a bidirectional prosthetic device control paradigm would fully capture the potential of upper extremity prostheses and could improve the quality of life of patients with amputations significantly.[35,44] Similar to recording efferent action potentials for motor control, several strategies have been used to provide sensory afferent feedback, including touch, pressure, proprioception, and finger position.[45] These stimulation techniques rely on similar strategies, previously discussed, and, therefore, face similar challenges. To overcome these challenges, RPNIs have been used to provide sensory afferent signals for sensory feedback from a prosthesis. RPNIs created on sensory and mixed nerves have been shown to restore proprioceptive sensations and cutaneous sensation in humans with upper limb amputations.[45,46] In addition, dermal-based sensory RPNIs that consist of de-epithelialized skin grafts reinnervated by residual sensory peripheral nerves have shown feasibility in transducing compound sensory nerve action potentials similar to native skin.[47]

In a step toward integrating sensory and motor signals, the composite RPNI (C-RPNI) has been developed.[48] It consists of a segment of free dermal and free muscle graft secured around a sensorimotor nerve. In rats, it has shown capability in transducing efferent motor action potentials to CMAPs with high SNRs and facilitating proximal CNSAPs with stimulation of the dermal component.[48] Through its ability to amplify efferent motor signals while simultaneously providing afferent sensory feedback, C-RPNIs hold promise as an interface for enabling the ideal neuroprosthetic control strategy.

SUMMARY

RPNIs transduce efferent motor action potentials to high-amplitude CMAPs with high SNRs, specificity, reliability, and stability and can be used to control a prosthetic hand with multiple degrees of freedom. They have been demonstrated to provide long-term stability with minimal needs for recalibration and have a safe clinical profile. Furthermore, RPNIs can be used to restore sensory feedback in upper limb amputations to allow closed loop neural control of a prosthesis and a more functional and natural prosthetic device experience. In doing so, RPNIs have revolutionized the potential of neuroprosthetic control of the upper extremity and created a more intuitive and enhanced experience for patients. Future studies remain to be performed that compare RPNIs as a prosthetic device control strategy to other existing techniques to accurately determine which method is most useful for different-level and different-limb amputations. Nevertheless, it has opened the door for significant advancements in the field of prosthetic technology and brings us one step closer to developing the ideal prosthetic experience and improving the quality of life of individuals living with amputations.

CLINICS CARE POINTS

- The regenerative peripheral nerve interface (RPNI) is a neuroprosthetic control strategy that transduces signals from residual peripheral nerves with high specificity and signal-to-noise ratios.
- RPNIs of the upper extremity have been performed in humans to enable intuitive control of an artificial hand and to execute finger movements.
- RPNIs can be used to transduce efferent motor signals and afferent sensory signals for enhanced prosthetic device control and user experience.
- To optimize functional restoration following limb loss, RPNIs should be created on all nerves and nerve fascicles responsible for upper limb hand function.

- Because electrodes interface directly with muscle in RPNIs, iatrogenic injury that occurs when electrodes directly interface with peripheral nerves is avoided.
- As individual fascicles can be used to create RPNIs, selective and specific prosthetic device control to support multiple degrees of freedom is possible leading to a more enhanced and intuitive experience compared to current neuroprosthetic control strategies.

ACKNOWLEDGMENTS

The authors would like to thank Dr Philip P. Vu and Alex Vaskov from the University of Michigan Neuromuscular Lab for their assistance with the included video in this article.

DISCLOSURE

There are no commercial or financial conflicts of interest and no funding sources for all authors for the work presented in this article.

SUPPLEMENTARY DATA

Supplementary data related to this article can be found online at https://doi.org/10.1016/j.hcl.2021.04.005.

REFERENCES

1. Yildiz KA, Shin AY, Kaufman KR. Interfaces with the peripheral nervous system for the control of a neuroprosthetic limb: a review. J Neuroeng Rehabil 2020; 17(1):43.
2. Uellendahl J. Myoelectric versus body-powered upper-limb prostheses: a clinical perspective. J Prosthetics Orthotics 2017;29(4S):25 9.
3. Kubiak CA, Kemp SWP, Cederna PS. Regenerative peripheral nerve interface for management of postamputation neuroma. JAMA Surg 2018;153(7):681–2.
4. Gaine WJ, Smart C, Bransby-Zachary M. Upper limb traumatic amputees. Review of prosthetic use. J Hand Surg Br 1997;22(1):73–6.
5. Østlie K, Lesjø IM, Franklin RJ, et al. Prosthesis use in adult acquired major upper-limb amputees: patterns of wear, prosthetic skills and the actual use of prostheses in activities of daily life. Disabil Rehabil Assist Technol 2012;7(6):479–93.
6. Kung TA, Bueno RA, Alkhalefah GK, et al. Innovations in prosthetic interfaces for the upper extremity. Plast Reconstr Surg 2013;132(6):1515–23.
7. Mohammadi A, Lavranos J, Zhou H, et al. A practical 3D-printed soft robotic prosthetic hand with multi-articulating capabilities. PLoS One 2020;15(5): e0232766.

8. Godfrey SB, Zhao KD, Theuer A, et al. The SoftHand Pro: Functional evaluation of a novel, flexible, and robust myoelectric prosthesis. PLoS One 2018; 13(10):e0205653.

9. Ngan CGY, Kapsa RMI, Choong PFM. Strategies for neural control of prosthetic limbs: from electrode interfacing to 3D printing. Materials (Basel) 2019; 12(12):1927.

10. Togo S, Murai Y, Jiang Y, et al. Development of an sEMG sensor composed of two-layered conductive silicone with different carbon concentrations. Sci Rep 2019;9(1):13996.

11. Schwartz AB, Cui XT, Weber DJ, et al. Brain-controlled interfaces: movement restoration with neural prosthetics. Neuron 2006;52(1):205–20.

12. Salisbury DB, Parsons TD, Monden KR, et al. Brain-computer interface for individuals after spinal cord injury. Rehabil Psychol 2016;61(4):435–41.

13. Lebedev MA, Nicolelis MA. Brain-machine interfaces: from basic science to neuroprostheses and neurorehabilitation. Physiol Rev 2017;97(2):767–837.

14. Bockbrader MA, Francisco G, Lee R, et al. Brain computer interfaces in rehabilitation medicine. PM R 2018;10(9 Suppl 2):S233–43.

15. Burns A, Adeli H, Buford JA. Brain-computer interface after nervous system injury. Neuroscientist 2014;20(6):639–51.

16. Dietrich D, Lang R, Bruckner D, et al. Limitations, possibilities and implications of brain-computer interfaces. 3rd International Conference on Human System Interaction, 2010. p. 722-6. Available at: https://ieeexplore.ieee.org/document/5514488.

17. Yanagisawa T, Hirata M, Saitoh Y, et al. Real-time control of a prosthetic hand using human electrocorticography signals. J Neurosurg 2011;114(6):1715–22.

18. Yanagisawa T, Hirata M, Saitoh Y, et al. Electrocorticographic control of a prosthetic arm in paralyzed patients. Ann Neurol 2012;71(3):353–61.

19. del Valle J, Navarro X. Interfaces with the peripheral nerve for the control of neuroprostheses. Int Rev Neurobiol 2013;109:63–83.

20. Thomp0son CH, Zoratti MJ, Langhals NB, et al. Regenerative electrode interfaces for neural prostheses. Tissue Eng B Rev 2016;22(2):125–35.

21. Lago N, Ceballos D, Rodríguez FJ, et al. Long term assessment of axonal regeneration through polyimide regenerative electrodes to interface the peripheral nerve. Biomaterials 2005;26(14):2021–31.

22. Urbanchek MG, Kung TA, Frost CM, et al. Development of a Regenerative Peripheral Nerve Interface for Control of a Neuroprosthetic Limb. Biomed Res Int 2016;2016:5726730.

23. Hopkins PM. Skeletal muscle physiology. Contin Educ Anaesth Crit Care Pain 2006;6(1):1–6.

24. Kung TA, Langhals NB, Martin DC, et al. Regenerative peripheral nerve interface viability and signal transduction with an implanted electrode. Plast Reconstr Surg 2014;133(6):1380–94.

25. Santosa KB, Oliver JD, Cederna PS, et al. Regenerative peripheral nerve interfaces for prevention and management of neuromas. Clin Plast Surg 2020; 47(2):311–21.

26. Dumont NA, Bentzinger CF, Sincennes MC, et al. Satellite cells and skeletal muscle regeneration. Compr Physiol 2015;5(3):1027–59.

27. Woo SL, Urbanchek MG, Cederna PS, et al. Revisiting nonvascularized partial muscle grafts: a novel use for prosthetic control. Plast Reconstr Surg 2014;134(2):344e–6e.

28. Frost CM, Ursu DC, Flattery SM, et al. Regenerative peripheral nerve interfaces for real-time, proportional control of a Neuroprosthetic hand. J Neuroeng Rehabil 2018;15(1):108.

29. Urbanchek MGW B, Baghmanli Z, Sugg KB, et al. Long-term stability of regenerative peripheral nerve interfaces (RPNI). Plast Reconstr Surg 2011; 128(4S):88–9.

30. Langhals NB, Woo SL, Moon JD, et al. Electrically stimulated signals from a long-term Regenerative Peripheral Nerve Interface. Conf Proc IEEE Eng Med Biol Soc 2014;2014:1989–92.

31. Irwin ZT, Schroeder KE, Vu PP, et al. Chronic recording of hand prosthesis control signals via a regenerative peripheral nerve interface in a rhesus macaque. J Neural Eng 2016;13(4):046007.

32. Vu PP, Irwin ZT, Bullard AJ, et al. Closed-loop continuous hand control via chronic recording of regenerative peripheral nerve interfaces. IEEE Trans Neural Syst Rehabil Eng 2018;26(2):515–26.

33. Vu PP, Vaskov AK, Irwin ZT, et al. A regenerative peripheral nerve interface allows real-time control of an artificial hand in upper limb amputees. Sci Transl Med 2020;12(533):eaay2857.

34. Dweiri YM, Eggers TE, Gonzalez-Reyes LE, et al. Stable detection of movement intent from peripheral nerves: chronic study in dogs. Proc IEEE 2017; 105(1):50–65.

35. Davis TS, Wark HA, Hutchinson DT, et al. Restoring motor control and sensory feedback in people with upper extremity amputations using arrays of 96 microelectrodes implanted in the median and ulnar nerves. J Neural Eng 2016;13(3):036001.

36. Ortiz-Catalan M, Mastinu E, Sassu P, et al. Self-contained neuromusculoskeletal arm prostheses. N Engl J Med 2020;382(18):1732–8.

37. Sahin M, Haxhiu MA, Durand DM, et al. Spiral nerve cuff electrode for recordings of respiratory output. J Appl Physiol (1985) 1997;83(1):317–22.

38. Struijk JJ, Thomsen M, Larsen JO, et al. Cuff electrodes for long-term recording of natural sensory information. IEEE Eng Med Biol Mag 1999;18(3):91–8.

39. Kuiken TA, Barlow AK, Hargrove L, et al. Targeted muscle reinnervation for the upper and lower extremity. Tech Orthop 2017;32(2):109–16.

40. Morgan EN, Kyle Potter B, Souza JM, et al. Targeted muscle reinnervation for transradial amputation: description of operative technique. Tech Hand Up Extrem Surg 2016;20(4):166–71.

41. Cheesborough JE, Smith LH, Kuiken TA, et al. Targeted muscle reinnervation and advanced prosthetic arms. Semin Plast Surg 2015;29(1):62–72.

42. Hargrove LJ, Miller LA, Turner K, et al. Myoelectric pattern recognition outperforms direct control for transhumeral amputees with targeted muscle reinnervation: a randomized clinical trial. Sci Rep 2017;7(1):13840.

43. Loeb GE. Taking control of prosthetic arms. JAMA 2009;301(6):670–1.

44. Tan DW, Schiefer MA, Keith MW, et al. A neural interface provides long-term stable natural touch perception. Sci Transl Med 2014;6(257):257ra138.

45. Nghiem BT, Sando IC, Gillespie RB, et al. Providing a sense of touch to prosthetic hands. Plast Reconstr Surg 2015;135(6):1652–63.

46. Vu P, Lu C, Vaskov A, et al. Restoration of proprioceptive and cutaneous sensation using Regenerative Peripheral Nerve Interfaces (RPNIs) in humans with upper-limb amputations. Plast Reconstr Surg Glob Open 2020;8(4 Suppl):65.

47. Sando ICG, Gregory J, Ursu DC, et al. Dermal-Based peripheral nerve interface for transduction of sensory feedback. Plast Reconstr Surg 2015; 136(4S):19–20.

48. Svientek SR, Ursu DC, Cederna PS, et al. Fabrication of the Composite Regenerative Peripheral Nerve Interface (C-RPNI) in the Adult Rat. J Vis Exp 2020; 25(156). 10.3791/60841.

The Agonist-Antagonist Myoneural Interface

Matthew J. Carty, MD[a],*, Hugh M. Herr, PhD[b]

KEYWORDS

• Agonist-antagonist myoneural interface • Amputation • Proprioception • Prostheses

KEY POINTS

- The agonist-antagonist myoneural interface (AMI) comprises innervated muscles that are biomechanically linked to recapitulate normal muscle-tendon agonist-antagonist dynamics, and a neural control architecture that electronically interfaces the linked muscle tendons to a powered external prosthesis.
- When incorporated into a limb amputation procedure, AMIs have the potential to augment volitional control of prostheses, preserve musculotendinous proprioception, and prevent residual limb atrophy.
- AMIs may be constructed from natively innervated or regenerative muscle units.
- To date, AMI construction has been applied to elective lower and upper extremity amputations as well as to lower extremity residual limb revision procedures.

INTRODUCTION

Profound changes are occurring in the realm of limb amputation. Once regarded as a form of surgical failure, amputation increasingly is being reframed as a reconstructive procedure—one with far more ambitious goals than those espoused in the past.[1] Whereas the prior aim of amputation largely was limited to providing a stable, padded residuum, current strategies have expanded expectations to include freedom from pain, high-fidelity control, neurosensory interfacing, and restoration of proprioceptive and cutaneous afferents. Fortunately, novel surgical approaches have been introduced over the past several years to meet these goals—among them, the agonist-antagonist myoneural interface (AMI). The AMI is a surgical construct and neuroprosthetic interfacing strategy designed to preserve or restore limb and joint proprioception, augment volitional control of adapted prostheses, and prevent or reverse limb atrophy. This article presents the authors' experience to date with the

development and implementation of the AMI in the setting of extremity amputation.

CONTEXT

Proprioception is the perception or awareness of the relative spatial positioning of one's body parts and the amount of force exerted on the environment.[2] Sometimes referred to as "the sixth sense," proprioception is critical to dexterity, joint stability, and mobile adaptation.[3] Although proprioceptive sensation has been ascribed to a symphony of mediators in human beings, the primary drivers appear to be muscle spindle fibers and Golgi tendon organs intrinsic to normal muscle-tendon architecture.[4] It is the stimulation of these structures, with the activation of dynamic agonist-antagonist muscle-tendon pairs in the intact body, that primarily establishes a neural loop between the peripheral and central nervous systems that, in turn, forms the basis for natural sensations of joint movement and load.[5]

The standard approach to amputation, however, disrupts dynamic agonist-antagonist muscle

a Division of Plastic Surgery, Brigham and Women's Hospital, Boston, MA, USA; b Center for Extreme Bionics, MIT Media Lab, Massachusetts Institute of Technology, 75 Amherst Street, Cambridge, MA 02139, USA
* Corresponding author: Division of Plastic Surgery, 1153 Centre Street, Jamaica Plain, MA 02130.
E-mail address: mcarty@bwh.harvard.edu

Hand Clin 37 (2021) 435–445
https://doi.org/10.1016/j.hcl.2021.04.006
0749-0712/21/© 2021 Elsevier Inc. All rights reserved.

relationships, resulting in isometric contraction of effector muscles with attempted phantom joint movement without compensatory stretch of their antagonist pairs. The resulting discordant neural milieu often produces aberrant phantom limb sensation that may contribute to the development of phantom pain.

The potential value of preserving proprioception in the setting of limb amputation initially was recognized through the development of the technique of cineplasty. First credited to Vanghetti[6] in 1898, the notion of cineplasty in its original form involved the construction of muscle loops or tubes covered with skin grafts to control adapted extremity prostheses. This loop design was further adapted by Sauerbruch[7] in 1916 to incorporate the use of "both protagonist and antagonist muscles to give physiologically correct control." Cineplasty achieved a moderate degree of popularity in the United States in the early 1950s, but its application largely was limited to the military population and never achieved widespread adoption due to issues with skin irritation, infection and muscle fatigue. As recently as 1998, proponents of cineplasty forecast the possibility of linking an adapted prosthetic device to a "cineplastized muscle's own proprioceptive receptors [in order to] provide feedback information about the prosthesis' state"[8]; however, an effective means of achieving a true, dynamic agonist-antagonist muscle-tendon unit coupled to a biomechanical device had yet to be described.

CONCEPT AND FOUNDATIONAL SCIENCE

The AMI represents an alternative vision to the loop cineplastic approach of agonist-antagonist coupling that exploits modern surgical techniques and neuroprosthetic interfacing to achieve enhanced prosthetic controllability and proprioceptive percepts. In contrast to cineplasty, the AMI approach does not seek to physically attach muscle-tendon units to an external prosthesis in order to complete the agonist-antagonist neuromechanical loop; rather, the AMI approach connects agonist-antagonist muscle-tendon units within the biological residuum and then bidirectionally communicates and interprets these tissue dynamics to an external prosthesis using sensors, stimulators and a control system. Because there does not exist direct physical loading between an external prosthesis and an agonist-antagonist muscle pair, the AMI approach mitigates the cineplastic issues of skin irritation, infection, and muscle fatigue.

The core notion of the AMI tissue construct is that a primary effector muscle (the agonist) is biomechanically linked in series to a counter-muscle (the antagonist) within the amputated residuum, such that contraction of the agonist results in simultaneous proportional stretch of the antagonist. Triggering of the agonist and/or antagonist may occur either through volitional, neural activation or via commanded means, including functional electrical stimulation (FES) from prosthetic processors. The stress and strain resulting from this dynamic relationship cause simultaneous stretch of the muscle spindle fibers and Golgi tendon organs within the agonist and antagonist muscle tendons, resulting in activation of both afferent and efferent neural pathways that recapitulate those of a natural biological system (**Fig. 1**). The specificity of agonist and antagonist muscle function imbues an individual AMI with the ability to serve as a proxy for a single lost or compromised joint; therefore, multiple AMIs have the potential to control multiple degrees of freedom within an external prosthesis.

When healthy, innervated, vascularized agonist-antagonist muscles with discrete, innate functionality are available, they may be redirected and biomechanically linked to enable the construction of native AMIs.[9,10] When such tissues are not available, however, they may be constructed de novo via techniques, including targeted muscle reinnervation (TMR) and/or regenerative peripheral nerve interface (RPNI) creation, and subsequently coapted via a passive material, such as tendon, thereby enabling the construction of regenerative AMIs (**Fig. 2**).

Preclinical studies of native AMI architecture provided the first proof of concept evidence regarding the validity of this reconstructive concept. Initial murine investigations demonstrated muscle stretch and integrated electroneurography (ENG) profiles for native AMIs to be similar to those of intact, uninjured agonist-antagonist hindlimb muscle dyads. Furthermore, the preservation of native neural loops was evidenced via the successful elicitation of antagonist muscle spindle fiber activation with agonist contraction.[11] Subsequent studies of native AMI construction in both below-knee amputation (BKA) and above-knee amputation (AKA) scenarios in larger caprine models demonstrated intact coupled motion of ankle and knee constructs, respectively, via both artificial muscle stimulation and direct mechanical manipulation.[12]

Validation of the regenerative approach to AMI construction was undertaken in parallel and demonstrated similarly promising results. Investigations in which single-stage AMI construction was performed via linked RPNI creation in a murine model evidenced coupled motion and

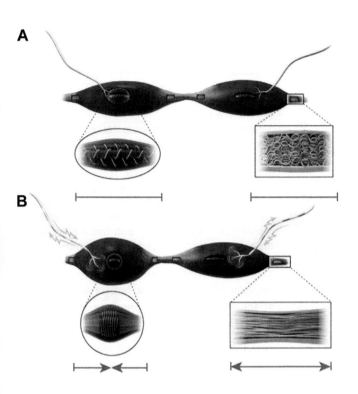

Fig. 1. AMI conceptual illustration. (*A*) Coapted agonist and antagonist muscle pair at rest, with quiescent muscle spindle fibers (*left*) and Golgi tendon organ (*right*). (*B*) Musculotendinous afferents along native neural pathways are produced when contraction of the agonist stretches the linked antagonist (or vice versa), causing activation of muscle spindle fibers and Golgi tendon organs.

physiologically relevant strains in all regenerative AMIs as well as the generation of graded electromyography (EMG) and ENG signals with construct stimulation.[13] Furthermore, follow-up murine studies in which 2-stage AMI construction was undertaken via RPNI creation during a first-stage surgery followed by AMI construct creation during a second-stage surgery (as would be required in a residual limb revision scenario) demonstrated similarly intact construct motion, afferent and efferent signaling, and force production. An additional serendipitous finding of this investigation was significant reversal of single RPNI muscle atrophy following AMI agonist-antagonist coaptation during the second-stage surgery.[14]

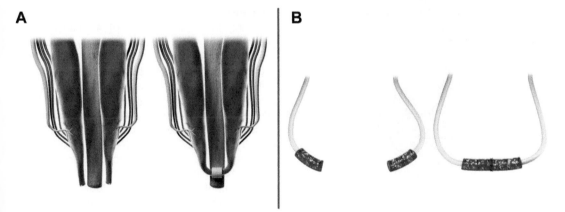

Fig. 2. Variations on AMI construction. (A) Native AMI design in which innervated, vascularized muscles with intended function are present. In this scenario, the distal ends of constituent agonist and antagonist muscles (left) may be simply redirected and coapted (right). (B) Regenerative AMI design, in which agonist and/or antagonist components must be created de novo. In this scenario, initial construction of innervated, vascularized muscle units first must be performed via TMR and/or RPNI techniques (left). Subsequent coaptation of regenerative units (right) may be performed as a second stage once innervation has been confirmed.

CLINICAL IMPLEMENTATION AND SURGICAL TECHNIQUES

The first human implementation of AMI construction was performed in 2016 in a modified BKA procedure that subsequently has been named the Ewing amputation. In this operation, 2 native AMIs were constructed; the first, composed of the tibialis anterior and lateral gastrocnemius, served as a tibiotalar joint emulator, whereas the second, composed of the peroneus longus and tibialis posterior, served as a subtalar joint emulator. Construction of each AMI was aided via the utilization of the patient's tarsal tunnels as spare parts, which were secured to anterior tibia using suture anchors and provided lubricious gliding mechanisms to which the constituent muscles were coapted (**Fig. 3**). Tensioning of each AMI construct was set to approximate normal

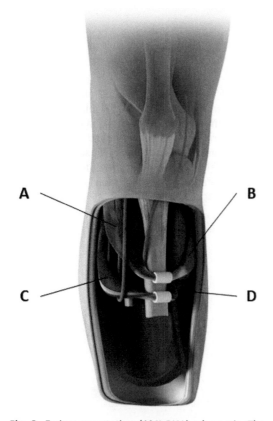

Fig. 3. Ewing amputation (AMI BKA) schematic. The upper AMI serves as the tibiotalar joint emulator and is composed of the (A) tibialis anterior and (B) lateral gastrocnemius, which is redirected around the posterior aspect of the limb to enter the AMI medially. The lower AMI serves as the subtalar joint emulator and is composed of the (C) peroneus longus and (D) tibialis posterior.

physiologic agonist-antagonist relationships, and radiopaque tantalum beads were inserted into each construct in order to facilitate noninvasive visualization of coapted motion in the postoperative period. Closure was performed via standard soleus myoplasty and approximation of soft tissue envelope edges.[15]

Since 2016, the Ewing amputation subsequently has been performed on 25 lower extremities in 22 patients under Partners institutional review board (IRB) Protocol 2014p001379. The original surgical technique has been modified slightly to include creation of a tibial periosteal overlay to protect the tarsal tunnel coaptation points and subfascial dissection of the posterior soft tissue envelope in order to augment skin perfusion. The most notable alteration, however, has been the incorporation of TMR and/or RPNI construction for neuroma prophylaxis of sensory nerve termini at the time of amputation; currently, the authors' practice is to ablate 5 distal nerves with significant cutaneous territories (tibial, superficial peroneal, deep peroneal, medial sural, and saphenous) via these techniques at the same time as performing AMI construction.

The authors' experience with the Ewing amputation has also informed the development of a modified approach to AKA, first performed in 2018 under Partners IRB Protocol 2014p001379. In this procedure, native AMIs are constructed for the tibiotalar and subtalar joints using the same muscle pairs as in the Ewing amputation; these are complemented, however, by the additional construction of a knee joint AMI composed of the rectus femoris and lateral head of the biceps femoris.[16] The tibiotalar and subtalar AMI muscles are recruited via isolation and mobilization of their discrete neurovascular pedicles—in essence, requiring the establishment of 4 neurovascular muscle island flaps that subsequently are configured circumferentially around the distal thigh musculature (**Fig. 4**). Tarsal tunnel recruitment is utilized for the 2 lower AMIs, as in the Ewing amputation, but provision of a gliding canal for the knee AMI is accomplished via utilization of ankle retinaculum or discarded muscle fascia.

AMI construction also has been incorporated into the design of novel approaches to modified upper extremity amputation at both the below-elbow amputation and above-elbow amputation (AEA) level under Partners IRB Protocol 2018p001893. In the former, AMI emulators for thumb interphalangeal joint flexion/extension, composite digital flexion/extension, and wrist flexion/extension are constructed via pairing of the flexor pollicis longus/extensor pollicis longus, flexor digitorum superficialis/extensor digitorum

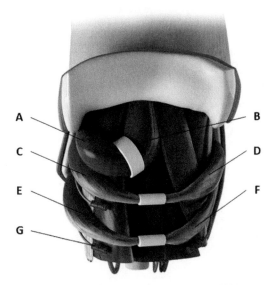

Fig. 4. AKA AMI schematic. The uppermost AMI serves as the knee joint emulator and is composed of the (A) lateral head of the biceps femoris and (B) rectus femoris. The middle AMI serves as the tibiotalar joint emulator and is composed of the (C) tibialis anterior and (D) lateral gastrocnemius. The lowermost AMI serves as the subtalar joint emulator and is composed of the (E) peroneus longus and (F) tibialis posterior. (G) Distal sensory nerve RPNI construct.

communis, and flexor carpi radialis/extensor carpi radialis brevis, respectively; in lieu of tarsal tunnels, the extensor retinaculum is utilized as a pulley stabilization platform over the distal end of the bony residuum.[17] In the single AEA procedure performed to date, a native AMI emulator for elbow flexion/extension was constructed utilizing pairing of the long head of the biceps and long head of the triceps. A regenerative AMI emulator for wrist flexion/extension was constructed using the short head of the biceps and lateral head of the triceps, because the patient had previously undergone TMR of the median and radial nerves to these sites. Pulley sites were created de novo in this case utilizing acellular dermal matrix (ADM) affixed to the epimysium of the distal residual limb myoplasty[18] (**Fig. 5**).

Most recently, AMI construction has been applied to the revision of previously amputated lower extremities at both the BKA and AKA level under Partners IRB Protocols 2017p000685 and 2019p001681. In the setting of BKA revision, sufficient musculature typically remains in the residual limb to enable the creation of native AMIs via techniques similar to those employed in a Ewing amputation; the notable exception, however, is that tarsal tunnels are not available for pulley construction, requiring substitution of ADM canals[19] (**Fig. 6**). AKA level revision obligatorily requires a combination of native (knee) and regenerative (tibiotalar and subtalar) AMI construction techniques due to the loss of predictable sciatic nerve organization other than gross division of the common peroneal and tibial nerve branches. In this scenario, the authors have pursued a 2-stage approach consisting of initial fascicular splitting of the sciatic nerve and multiple RPNI construction, followed by EMG interrogation of RPNIs approximately 3 months to 6 months later and subsequent surgical coupling of the functionally specific regenerative units into AMI constructs as a follow-up procedure. This regenerative revision procedure has been coupled with simultaneous

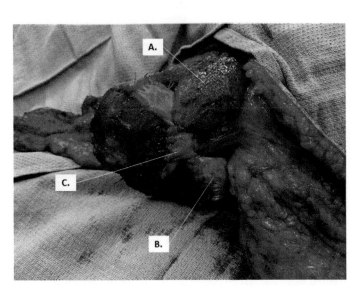

Fig. 5. AEA AMI clinical photograph. Native elbow joint AMI composed of the (A) long head of biceps and (B) lateral head of triceps. (C) ADM canal and distal platform to stabilize AMI pivot point.

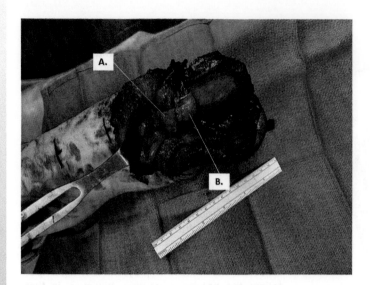

Fig. 6. AMI construction in BKA revision scenario. (A) Tibiotalar joint AMI. (B) Subtalar joint AMI.

placement of an experimental transfemoral osseointegrated implant (eOPRA device, Integrum, San Francisco, California) in order to maximize downstream functional potential and volitional control[20] (**Fig. 7**).

OUTCOMES

To date, a majority of amputation procedures incorporating AMIs have been performed in elective BKA or AKA scenarios; as a result, the preponderance of outcomes data collected pertains to

these procedures. These outcomes are summarized.

Clinical Parameters

A total of 25 modified BKA procedures and 4 modified AKA procedures have been performed to date in a total of 26 patients. Average operative times for modified BKA and AKA procedures have been 340 minutes ± 63 minutes and 562 minutes ± 120 minutes, respectively. Average length of stay for BKA patients has been

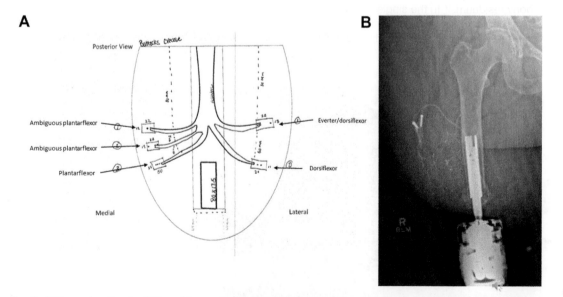

Fig. 7. AMI construction in AKA revision scenario, including placement of eOPRA device. (*A*) Schematic diagram depicting construction of multiple RPNIs from sciatic nerve and ultimate reinnervated function determined via EMG. Appropriate agonist and antagonist pairs subsequently were coapted in a second-stage procedure. (*B*) Plain radiograph depicting eOPRA device and implanted electrode system connected to AMI tissue constructs.

5.4 days ± 1.6 days, whereas that of AKA patients has been 14.5 days ± 10.1 days. The clinical parameters pertaining to both categories of patients are summarized in **Table 1**.[21]

Complications

Among the modified BKA population, 3 (12%) operative limbs have demonstrated minor wound healing issues, whereas 4 (16%) have demonstrated major wound healing issues requiring operative intervention. Three (12%) BKA limbs have demonstrated minor infections requiring postoperative oral antibiotic therapy. Eight (32%) BKA limbs have required operative revision for soft tissue modification, osteophyte excision, neuroma ablation, and/or suture anchor removal. Among the modified AKA population, 2 patients (50%) have demonstrated significant necrosis of their soft tissue envelopes requiring operative débridement and revision closure with split-thickness skin grafts. No additional complications in either patient cohort have been reported to date.[21]

Agonist-Antagonist Myoneural Interface Function

Subjective reports of the degree of AMI activation and excursion by both patients and providers have been ranked uniformly as good (46%) or very good (54%) in serial clinical examinations for up to 3 years postoperatively. Objective interrogation of AMI constructs via serial ultrasound studies have demonstrated persistent preservation of coupled motion in all modified BKA and AKA patients over time, with a mean excursion of 4.3 mm ± 1.2 mm across muscle coaptation sites that has remained stable for up to 33 months following amputation.[21] Furthermore, assessments of antagonist muscle fascicle strain with agonist muscle contraction have exhibited statistically significant differences between modified BKA patients and standard BKA controls[22] as well as between modified AKA patients and standard AKA controls.[16] Fascicle strain assessments between modified BKA and modified AKA patients were noted to be comparable, suggesting a relative equivalency of excursion dynamics across both experimental groups.

Limb Morphology

As referenced in **Table 1**, serial circumferential measurements obtained over time have demonstrated 94.3% ± 4.8% and 100.6% ± 5.4% preservation of residual limb volume in modified BKA and modified AKA patients, respectively, that has persisted for up to 36 months postoperatively. The etiology of this preserved limb bulk most likely is due to unconscious activation of constituent AMI musculature with regular ambulation, resulting in muscle volume maintenance and, in some cases, hypertrophy. This relative stability in limb

---

Table 1
Agonist-antagonist myoneural interface lower extremity amputation study subject clinical parameters

Measure	Agonist-Antagonist Myoneural Interface Below-Knee Amputations		Agonist-Antagonist Myoneural Interface Above-Knee Amputations	
	Total/Mean	SD	Total/Mean	SD
Total patients	22	—	4	—
Total limbs	25	—	4	—
Age (y)	41.3	12.5	40.6	19
Gender (% M/F)	59/41	—	25/75	—
BMI (kg/m²)	27.7	5.3	23.1	8.2
Operative time (min)	340	63	562	120
Fluids (mL)	1536	603	2125	299
EBL (mL)	86	74	213	193
UOP (mL)	672	330	1078	454
LOS (d)	5.4	1.6	14.5	10.1
Drain removal (d)	12.3	3.4	11.5	6.4
Prosthesis fitting (d)	67.8	33.1	74.3	28.3
Volume preservation (%)	94.3	4.8	100.6	5.4

Abbreviations: BMI, body mass index; EBL, estimated blood loss; F, female; LOS, length of stay; M, male; UOP, urine output.

morphology has translated to subjective patient reports of infrequent requirements for socket refitting once postoperative swelling has resolved, with a majority of patients having unchanged interfaces for at least 12 months to 18 months.[23]

Pain

All patients who have undergone modified BKA or AKA procedures have demonstrated a complete wean from narcotic medications in the postoperative period, with an average wean time of 58 days and a range of 4 days to 189 days. The upper end of this range is due at least in part to a subset of intervention patients who were on chronic opioid medications for many years prior to surgery and thus required extended wean protocols due to concerns about potential withdrawal; 38% of patients who have undergone these procedures report residual limb pain; of these, 78% report such pain to be rare or occasional and are managed via over-the-counter medications or nonpharmacologically. Two patients who did not undergo initial sensory nerve ablation at the time of their amputation subsequently required TMR procedures to successfully address neuropathic residual limb pain; 29% of intervention patients report some degree of phantom limb pain, but all such patients report this pain to be rare.[21]

Rehabilitation

All modified BKA and AKA patients have progressed to standard prosthesis fitting following complete healing of their residual limbs at a mean interval of 67.8 days ± 33.1 days and 74.3 days ± 28.3 days, respectively (see **Table 1**), and universally report utilization of their prostheses for 10 hours to 12 hours per day. Furthermore, they have been assessed via a battery of validated rehabilitation metrics at standard time points throughout their clinical courses. Comparisons of functional status performed in the preoperative versus post-prosthesis periods have demonstrated improvements in the 10-m walking test (20% ± 40%), timed up and go test (12% ± 44%) figure-of-8 test (23% ± 41%), side step (58% ± 57%), functional reach test (16% ± 70%), 4-stair climb test (14% ± 49%), and 6-minute walking test (42% ± 93%).[24]

Patient-reported Outcomes Measurements

All modified BKA and AKA patients have been administered 3 validated patient-reported outcomes measurement instruments in the preoperative setting and at set intervals postoperatively (every 3 months for the first year and annually thereafter)—the EuroQol (EQ)-5D, the Lower Extremity Functional Scale (LEFS), and the Patient Reported Outcomes Measurement Information System (PROMIS)-57. Reporting at a mean postoperative interval of 15.9 months ± 5.3 months, respondents have demonstrated uniform improvements in all measured categories relative to baseline. Specifically, intervention patients have demonstrated improvements in the EQ-5D health scale (129% ± 229%) and LEFS overall score (170% ± 185%) as well as PROMIS-57 physical function (144% ± 141%), anxiety (−11% ± 44%), depression (−4% ± 62%), fatigue (−41% ± 27%), sleep disturbance (−13% ± 47%), social roles and activities (150% ± 136%), pain interference (−55% ± 33%), and pain intensity (−57% ± 50%).[21]

Sensory Feedback

Among modified BKA and AKA patients, 85% have reported significant phantom limb sensation following their procedures. A majority of patients report this phantom sensation to be anatomically correct in terms of position and proportion of their phantom limb, with specific territories of the phantom particularly present (**Fig. 8**). These patients typically state that their phantom limb sensation is augmented by activation of their AMI constructs, with many claiming an ability to "summon" or "telescope" their phantom limb with AMI motion. Furthermore, comparative studies have demonstrated significantly higher degrees of phantom limb sensation in AMI BKA patients versus standard BKA patients.[22]

Central Neuroplasticity

Functional neuroimaging of AMI BKA patients, standard BKA patients and patients without amputations has demonstrated that AMI BKA patients manifest functional activation of Brodmann area (BA) 3a, which traditionally is considered to be the nexus for proprioception in the central nervous system, in a manner similar to those with intact limbs; this is in contrast to patients with standard BKAs, who demonstrate diminished activation of this cortical region. Furthermore, AMI BKA patients have demonstrated enhanced functional sensorimotor connectivity and phantom sensation compared with standard BKA patients, evidenced via increased activation of areas in the medial frontal cortex, including BA3a, BA3b, BA4a, and BA4p. These results suggest that AMI construction has a measurable neuroplastic effect in reengaging sensory feedback and motor imagery functionality.[25]

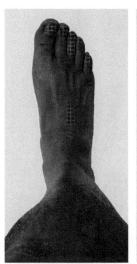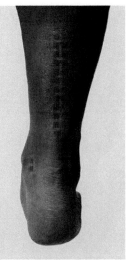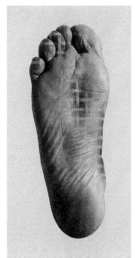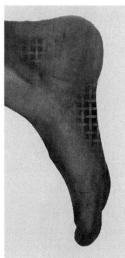

Fig. 8. Phantom limb sensation mapping in AMI BKA subject. Hatched areas depict regions of maximal phantom limb perception, as indicated by patient, in phantom dorsal foot, posterior leg, plantar foot and medial foot (left to right).

Linkage with Adapted Protheses

Patients who undergo modified amputations with AMI construction likely will achieve their maximal functional potential when their residual limb is coapted to an adapted prosthesis capable of interfacing with their unique surgical architecture. Toward this end, pilot investigations have been completed in which an experimental prosthetic leg with powered artificial tibiotalar and subtalar joints has been connected to the residual limb of a BKA AMI patient via both surface and percutaneous needle electrodes (**Fig. 9**). Compared with patients who underwent standard BKAs, the BKA AMI patient demonstrated markedly improved independent volitional control of joint position and impedance when linked to the experimental device as well as intuitive restoration of reflexive behaviors during various stages of the stair ascent and descent gait cycle. Furthermore, experiments in which FES was utilized in order to provide afferent proprioceptive feedback of joint torque resulted in markedly improved performance on torque control tasks in the BKA AMI patient that were not witnessed in standard BKA controls. Lastly, the BKA AMI patient demonstrated significant evidence of augmented embodiment with the adapted prosthesis, manifest through a variety of small behaviors including unconscious fidgeting of his mechanical foot while engaged in conversation as well as during interviews in which he stated, "I felt like I had a foot. I think that in just the short time I had it wired in and mounted to me it was quickly becoming a part of me."[26,27]

LIMITATIONS

Although the AMI appears to offer many advantages, it is not a true emulator of natural joint dynamics. In a normal, uninjured scenario, the agonist and antagonist muscles operating around an intact joint do not undergo loads exclusively via antagonistic muscle actions; in particular, they frequently undergo stretch due to forces arising from gravitation and inertia. The AMI agonist is capable only of experiencing these load conditions via volitional or external FES activation of its antagonist muscle partner; because both the agonist and antagonist muscles are innervated, this may result in an unnatural perception of antagonist activation by the person with amputation. Furthermore, the AMI necessarily reduces the mechanics of a given joint to an oversimplified architecture consisting of a single agonist and a single antagonist. The muscle dynamics that are witnessed in an intact joint, however, are characterized more frequently by the activation of several muscles with differential lines of action and, in turn, differential contraction/stretch profiles. Whether the AMI remains a close enough emulator of native joint dynamics remains unclear and will be the focus of ongoing research efforts.

SUMMARY AND FUTURE DIRECTIONS

The AMI is a novel surgical construct that appears to augment volitional motor control of adapted prostheses, preserve proprioception, and maintain residual limb volume when applied to an acute lower extremity amputation model. Investigations

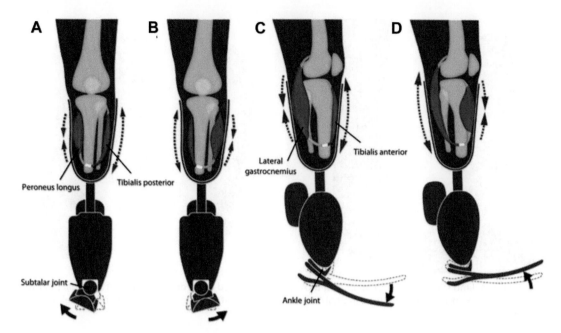

Fig. 9. Schematic depicting linkage of AMI BKA residual limb to experimental prosthesis. Surface and/or fine-needle electrodes transmit volitional activation of AMIs to powered limb, resulting in (*A*) eversion, (*B*) inversion, (*C*) plantarflexion, and (*D*) dorsiflexion.

to further validate the value of AMI construction in the setting of upper limb amputation and residual limb revision currently are under way, with pilot procedures of both of these scenarios already having been completed. Furthermore, AMI implementation also is being combined with the development of emerging technologies, including next-generation prostheses and osseointegrated implants specifically designed to interface with AMI surgical architecture. The authors look forward to sharing the results of these ongoing investigations in the future.

More broadly, AMI implementation figures into an emerging paradigm of functional limb restoration in which fundamental redesign of the peripheral nervous system and its effectors is possible. Currently, the use case for the AMI has been to optimize function and minimize pain in the scenario of limb loss; however, there is little reason to believe that similar value would not be achieved in the setting of partial limb injury, degenerative disease, and/or paralysis. Furthermore, AMI construction (either in isolation or in conjunction with other novel reconstructive procedures) potentially may be applied to scenarios in which the goal is to augment, rather than restore, human functionality—and thereby extend the potential capabilities beyond presently accepted norms. The authors are excited about exploring such possibilities in the coming years.

CLINICS CARE POINTS

- When performing limb amputation, consideration should be given by the care team to the potential benefits of incorporating AMI construction into the surgical plan
- AMI construction also should be regarded as an option when pursuing revision of residual limbs due to soft tissue breakdown or neuropathic pain

DISCLOSURE

Dr M.J. Carty and Dr H.M. Herr both currently receive grant income from the DARPA Haptix Program (W911NF-17-2-0043), CDMRP (PRORP-CTA OR160165A; PRORP-CTA OR170384; PRORP-CTA OR180114), Defense Medical Research and Development Program (W81XWH-19-1-0151), and the NIH (1R01HD097135-01). The authors have 2 submitted patents on the AMI and its application to prosthetic control.

Funded by: DOD. *Grant number(s):* CDMRP/ PRORP OR160165; CDMRP/PRORP OR170384; CDMRP/PRORP OR180114.

REFERENCES

1. Herr HM, Clites TR, Srinivasan SS, et al. Reinventing extremity amputation in the era of functional limb restoration. Ann Surg 2020;273(2):269–79.
2. Proske U, Gandevia SC. The proprioceptive senses: Their role in signaling body shape, body position and movement, and muscle force. Physiol Rev 2012;92:1651–97.
3. Riemann BL, Lephart SM. The sensorimotor system, part II: The role of proprioception in motor control and functional joint stability. J Athl Train 2002;37: 80–4.
4. Kandell ER, Schwartz JH, Jessell TM. Principles of neural science, vol. 4. New York: McGraw-Hill; 2013. p. 1414.
5. Ribot-Ciscar E, Roll JP. Ago-antagonist muscle spindle inputs contribute together to joint movement coding in man. Brain Res 1998;791:167–76.
6. Vanghetti G. Amputazioni: disaticolozioni e protesi. Florence: s.n.; 1898.
7. Sauerbruch F. Die Willkulich Bewegbare Kunstliche Hand. 1st edition. Berlin: Julious Springer-Verlag; 1916.
8. Weir RF. A century of the Sauerbruch-Lebsche-Vanghetti muscle cineplasty: the United States experience, vol. 7. Northwestern University Capabilities; 1998.
9. Herr HM, Riso RR, Song KW, et al,. Peripheral neural interface via nerve regeneration to distal tissues. 14/ 520,766 United States, October 22, 2014.
10. Herr HM, Clites TR, Maimon B, et al. Method and system for providing proprioceptive feedback and functionality mitigating limb pathology. 62/276,422 United States, January 24, 2019.
11. Clites TR, Carty MJ, Srinivasan S, et al. A murine model of a novel surgical architecture for proprioceptive muscle feedback and its potential application to control of advanced limb prostheses. J Neural Eng 2017;14:036002.
12. Clites TR, Carty MJ, Srinivasan SS, et al. Caprine models of the agonist-antagonist myoneural interface implemented at the above- and below-knee amputation levels. Plast Reconstr Surg 2019;144: 218e–29e.
13. Srinivasan SS, Carty MJ, Calvaresi PW, et al. On prosthetic control: A regenerative agonist-antagonist myoneural interface. Sci Robot 2017;2: eaan2971.
14. Srinivasan SS, Diaz M, Carty MJ, et al. Towards functional restoration for persons with limb amputation: A dual-stage implementation of regenerative agonist-antagonist myoneural interfaces. Sci Rep 2019;9:1981.
15. Clites TR, Herr HM, Srinivasan SS, et al. The Ewing amputation: The first human implementation of the agonist-antagonist myoneural interface. Plast Reconst Surg Glob Open 2018;6:e1997.
16. Srinivasan SS, Herr HM, Clites TR, et al. Agonist-antagonist myoneural interfaces in above-knee amputation preserve distal joint function and perception. Ann Surg 2021;273(3):e115–8.
17. Souza J, Potter BK, Tintle S, et al. Agonist-antagonist myoneural interface implementation in upper extremity amputation. 2021. Manuscript in process.
18. Souza J, Potter BK, Herr HM, et al. The first human implementation of regenerative agonist-antagonist myoneural interface construction in upper limb amputation. 2021. Manuscript in process.
19. Carty MJ, Berger L, Herr HM. The first implementation of agonist-antagonist myoneural interface construction in a below knee amputation revision. 2021. Manuscript in process.
20. Carty MJ, Branemark R, O'Donnell R, et al. Regenerative agonist-antagonist myoneural construction in an above knee amputation revision in conjunction with eOPRA device placement. 2021. Manuscript in process.
21. Carty MJ, Berger L, Landry T. Early clinical outcomes from lower extremity amputations incorporating AMI design. 2021. Manuscript in process.
22. Srinivasan SS, Gutierrez-Arango S, Teng AC, et al. Neural interfacing architecture enables enhanced residual limb functionality post amputation. Proc Natl Acad Sci U S A 2020;118(9). e2019555118.
23. Berger L, Beltran L, Weischoff G, et al. Limb morphology stability following modified BKA and AKA procedures incorporating agonist-antagonist myoneural interfaces. 2021. Manuscript in process.
24. Welch S, Berger L, Carty MJ. Rehabilitative outcomes of patients who have undergone lower extremity amputation incorporating AMI design. 2021. Manuscript in process.
25. Srinivasan SS, Tuckute G, Zou J, et al. Agonist-antagonist myoneural interface amputation preserves proprioceptive sensorimotor neurophysiology in lower limbs. Sci Transl Med 2020;12(573): eabc5926.
26. Clites TR, Carty MJ, Ullauri JB, et al. Proprioception from a neurally controlled lower-extremity prosthesis. Sci Transl Med 2018;10(443):eaap8373.
27. Rogers EA, Carney ME, Yeoh SH, et al. An ankle-foot prosthesis for rock climbing augmentation. IEEE Trans Neural Syst Rehabil Eng 2020;29:41–51.

Starfish Procedure

Andrew Jordan Grier, MD[a], Bryan J. Loeffler, MD[b,c],
Raymond Glenn Gaston, MD[b,c],*

KEYWORDS

- Amputation • Electromyographic signal • Myoelectric control • Prosthesis
- Interossei muscle transfer • Partial hand amputation • Ray resection

KEY POINTS

- Restoring functional outcomes following partial hand amputations remains a challenge, given the difficulties experienced by patients in completion of both fine motor and power grasp tasks.
- Myoelectric digital control in patients with partial hand amputations remains challenging due to the lack of availability of intuitive electromyographic (EMG) signals for prosthesis control.
- The Starfish Procedure allows for the transfer of functioning intrinsic musculature to create sources of EMG signals capable of individual digital control with a prosthesis. This novel transfer method allows for creation of high-quality signals with minimal myoelectric cross-talk.
- An advantage of the Starfish Procedure is that it does not require microsurgical techniques, and it is not a technically demanding procedure.
- The intuitive nature of the transfers performed allows for rapid prosthesis adoption and use by patients, which may allow for increased functional use and increased prosthesis utilization compared with historical controls.

 Video content accompanies this article at http://www.hand.theclinics.com.

INTRODUCTION

Despite a large armamentarium of reconstructive options, the management of partial hand amputations remains a challenging clinical scenario. Trauma at the level of the palm differs from that at the digit level due to the presence of the intrinsic hand musculature, which may undergo severe blunt injury, contamination, and resultant muscle necrosis due to extensive devitalization.[1] In addition, these injuries pose a significant risk to the deep and superficial palmar arches, as well as proximal portions of the common digital nerves, thereby threatening the neurovascular status of replanted tissues. Replantation following traumatic transmetacarpal amputation is often fraught with limitations in function and sensibility, resulting in fair or poor results in greater than 50% of patients in long-term follow-up series.[1,2] Despite the suboptimal functional outcomes observed, many patients report subjective satisfaction with their outcome and are able to return to work in some capacity.[1–3]

Similarly, results following replantation of multiple digits have demonstrated only modest overall improvements relative to amputation with respect to ultimate patient outcomes. In a recent review of more than 300 patients undergoing either replantation or revision amputation following single or multiple digit amputation, it was observed that those patients with either 2 digits or 3 or more digits amputated experienced significant improvements in DASH and PROMIS scores following replantation when one of the involved digits was the thumb.[4] However, when excluding the thumb, no significant improvements in patient-reported

[a] OrthoCarolina Hand Center, 1915 Randolph Road, Charlotte, NC 28207, USA; [b] Reconstructive Center for Lost Limbs, OrthoCarolina Hand Center, 1915 Randolph Road, Charlotte, NC 28207, USA; [c] Department of Orthopaedic Surgery, Atrium Healthcare, Charlotte, NC, USA
* Corresponding author. Reconstructive Center for Lost Limbs, OrthoCarolina Hand Center, 1915 Randolph Road, Charlotte, NC 28207.
E-mail address: Glenn.gaston@orthocarolina.com

Hand Clin 37 (2021) 447–455
https://doi.org/10.1016/j.hcl.2021.04.007

outcomes were observed with replantation of either 2 digits or 3 or more digits, suggesting that the outcomes following replantation of multiple nonthumb digits may not provide meaningful improvements in patient function compared with revision amputation. Salvage operations including heterotopic replantation and vascularized single or multiple toe transfers are options in certain clinical scenarios; however, these procedures frequently require advanced microsurgical techniques not available at some centers.[5,6] Although acceptable motion may be achieved following toe transfer, short- and intermediate-term outcomes demonstrate key pinch strength of only 41% to 70% of their uninjured hand.[7–9] Similarly, grip strength following toe transfer can be expected to reach only 26% of their contralateral hand, which is not sufficient for completion of many of the high-demand tasks performed by these patients.[9] The long-term results of salvage reconstructive procedures remain unpredictable as a result of the heterogeneity of injuries and quality of tissue available for transfer and may not be an appropriate solution for many patients.[10–12]

Partial resection of the hand has also gained favor as a treatment option for sarcomas when the ability to achieve negative microscopic margins is possible.[13,14] This approach allows for retention of well-functioning, disease-free digits without imparting added risk of local recurrence, which would be present if negative margins were unachievable. Prolonged vasopressor use, particularly norepinephrine, frequently results in peripheral vasoconstriction, which disproportionately affects the distal portions of the hand and feet.[15] The duration of exposure and dose of vasoactive agent may show an ultimate result in an unsalvageable degree of digital ischemia necessitating partial hand amputation.[16,17]

Prosthesis options for patients with partial hand or multiple digit amputations have historically provided unsatisfactory function relative to that of the patient's native digits due to multiple drawbacks including weight, durability, socket discomfort, and limited prehensile capabilities.[18,19] These limitations have resulted in rates of prosthesis rejection of greater than 30% in upper extremity amputees.[20–22] Currently available prostheses include passive, body-powered, and externally powered myoelectric devices. Of the available options, myoelectric devices are particularly appealing, as they allow for more advanced active prehensile function relative to their passive or body-powered counterparts, but they are limited by the low number of detectible myoelectric signals and typically require nonintuitive control. Advances in myoelectric prosthesis design provide for improved digital control; however, successful signal transmission is limited by the quality of surface electromyographic (EMG) signals captured at the patient-prosthesis interface.[23] The signal quality transmitted at the surface electrode interface is reliant on both the amplitude and relative clarity (absence of undesirable signals from adjacent muscle or myoelectric cross-talk) of signal generated by the underlying muscle.[23,24]

Myoelectric digital control in patients with partial hand amputations is challenging due to limitations in detecting desirable EMG signals for intuitive digital flexion and extension. These signals can come from either the intrinsic muscles of the hand or from the extrinsic flexors and extensors in the forearm. Aside from the first dorsal interosseous (DI) and hypothenar musculature, the EMG signals from other hand intrinsics are too weak to be detected by surface electrodes due to the small size of the signals and the distance between their muscle bellies and the skin. In addition, transducing myoelectric signals into individual digital control signals remains challenging due to the relatively small size and dense anatomy of the intrinsics at the level of the midpalm.[25] Composite digital control from the first dorsal interosseous or hypothenar muscles is typically nonintuitive, requiring patients to think about abduction of all digits to open the prosthetic hand and adduction of all digits to close the prosthetic hand. Most commercially available myoelectric hands contain 2 to 3 surface electrodes that obtain signals from intrinsic hand muscles or extrinsic (forearm) sources and generate either simultaneous hand-opening or simultaneous hand-closing movements in the myoelectric digits.[25,26] Forearm level sensors provide an alternative source of signal transmission; however, this interface also requires nonintuitive control patterns (ie, wrist flexion required for grasp and wrist extension for release functions).[27] Forearm level control also necessitates a prosthesis of added length and weight, which by design must traverse the wrist joint, thus limiting wrist mobility during prosthesis wear.

Based on the shortcomings noted in the currently used human-prosthesis EMG interfaces, the need for an improved means of control for commercially available myoelectric prostheses was identified. A cadaveric study was performed for metacarpophalangeal (MCP) level amputations in order to evaluate the feasibility of transferring the intrinsic muscles to a superficial location while maintaining their neurovascular pedicles. The goal of the transfers was to position an intrinsic muscle corresponding to each amputated digit, which would enable detection of intuitive EMG signals of sufficient quality to control commercially available myoelectric digits. From this initial cadaveric dissection, it was determined that it may be possible to use the available intrinsic hand musculature in a novel pattern to provide for a more favorable EMG signal profile and potentially allow intuitive, individual digital control with a prosthesis. The Starfish Procedure allows for creation of separate, anatomically insulated sources of signal for intuitive individual myoelectric digit control using a patient's available intrinsic musculature.[28] A thorough understanding of the anatomy of the remaining intrinsic musculature on an individual patient basis allows for thoughtful intrinsic muscle transfers that provide immediately available EMG signals for use in conjunction with currently available myoelectric prosthesis designs. The proposed transfers can be achieved without the use of microsurgery or other technically demanding surgical techniques, allowing for adaptation of the described techniques by treating surgeons without advanced microsurgical training.

INDICATIONS AND CONTRAINDICATIONS

Patients with amputations at or distal to the proximal interphalangeal (PIP) joint often have sufficient digital length to maintain useful grasp and hand function and do not require surgical reconstruction (**Fig. 1**). At times, these patients may benefit from digital prostheses. When amputations occur between the MCP and PIP joints, the functional capability of the digit is severely compromised. Typically, the digit is unable to meaningfully contribute to grasp. In order to enable prosthetic fitting, there must be roughly enough digit remaining on which to place a ring. If we estimate enough length with soft tissue covering to place a ring on the digit, we will salvage the digit in hopes of enabling use of a finger prosthesis. In dealing with multidigit amputations, this serves as a guide when we consider maintaining a digit versus

performing a more proximal level amputation and the Starfish Procedure.

Patients with nonreplantable partial hand amputations at, or distal to, the midmetacarpal level, with viable intrinsic hand musculature remaining, are considered suitable candidates for the Starfish Procedure. To date, causes leading to patients' index operations include trauma, deep soft tissue infection, local tissue ischemia (vasopressor-induced ischemia, acute vascular injury, chronic ischemia/gangrene), and limb-sparing oncologic resection (**Fig. 2**, Video 1). Contraindications to the procedure include acute replantable digits or partial hand amputations, insufficient intrinsic hand musculature to provide the requisite myoelectric signals, ongoing infection of the residual limb, cognitive impairment that limits the patient's ability to control a prosthesis, or an ipsilateral brachial plexus palsy or ulnar nerve palsy rendering the intrinsics paralyzed.

The Starfish Procedure can also be performed on a delayed basis following a partial hand amputation. In these cases, if the amputation is at or distal to the midmetacarpal level, then the intrinsic musculature is typically preserved and has sufficient bulk to function for prosthetic control. If the functional status of the interossei is in question, based on residual metacarpal length or soft tissue injury, then we will perform a formal EMG to ensure viability and function of the intrinsics before considering surgery. In cases of delayed Starfish Procedures, we attempt to obtain insurance authorization for the prosthesis before scheduling surgery, because the patient will not experience functional gain without acquiring a myoelectric, partial hand prosthesis.

SURGICAL TECHNIQUE

The patient is positioned supine on the operating table with the affected extremity on a radiolucent

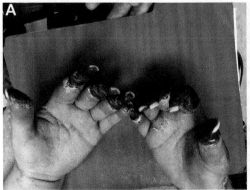
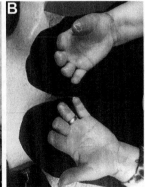
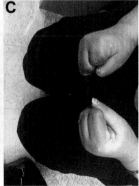

Fig. 1. (*A–C*) Necrotic sequelae of vasopressor-induced ischemia of the left and right hands. Figures B and C demonstrate healing following functional PIP level amputations of both hands.

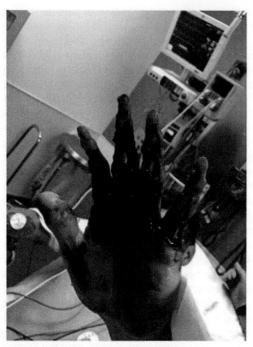

Fig. 2. A 53-year-old man who sustained a complete degloving to the nondominant left hand. After a discussion regarding groin flap coverage versus 4-finger Starfish Procedure the patient elected to proceed with amputation and Starfish transfers. The patient subsequently returned to work at a modified-duty level at 10 weeks postoperatively. At 6 months postoperatively the patient had returned to full duty driving a fork-lift without restrictions.

hand table extension. Either regional or general anesthesia is administered at the treating surgeons' discretion. The initial stages of the surgical dissection may vary based on the patient's underlying cause for presentation and may entail concomitant bony or soft tissue procedures before turning attention to muscle transfer.

One philosophic change has taken place in our management of acute multidigit replant cases. The classic teaching has been to prioritize thumb, followed by long, ring, small, and index finger in that order.[29] We still prioritize the thumb first but then consider the index finger as the next most importance. This change is because we have found it critical to have a sensate thumb-index pinch for performing fine motor activities such as writing, picking up a coin, etc. By using the Starfish Procedure for the ulnar 3 digits (when salvage is not possible) we can provide excellent grasp function for heavier demand activities. If a more central digit is replanted (or toe transferred), the available space for a prosthesis is compromised; and although patients can adequately perform tasks

requiring simple pinch, they struggle grasping objects of significant weight. In cases in which adequate length of the index finger cannot be maintained and the thumb has also lost length, heterotopic transfer of the remaining index finger to the thumb can be performed to provide additional length to the thumb (**Fig. 3**, Video 2).

Generally, the procedure begins with disarticulation of any remaining tissue of the involved rays at the MCP joint level to facilitate exposure of the intrinsic hand musculature. The exposure should be carried proximally by raising a dorsal full-thickness flap inclusive of the subcutaneous tissues and extrinsic extensor mechanism such that the involved metacarpals and interossei can be visualized to the level of the metacarpal base. The desired DI are then sharply elevated in an extraperiosteal fashion from their adjacent metacarpals. The DI are mobilized proximally until sufficient length for dorsal transfer has been achieved, with care taken to preserve their accompanying neurovascular pedicles, which enter the DI at roughly the level of the metacarpal metaphyseal flare. Each DI of interest must be carefully separated from the associated volar interossei (VI) of their respective webspace in order to avoid unintended transfer of VI tissue. This step is critical as the second, third, and fourth webspaces have 2 interossei, each controlling a different digit. For example, at the second webspace the first VI adducts the index finger, whereas the second DI abducts the long finger. Failure to separate these interossei will result in undesirable, conflicting signal transduction, which may prevent the intended means of digital control. After adequate mobilization of the interossei to be transferred is complete, transmetacarpal resection is performed on the involved rays using a microsagittal saw. Attention should be paid to careful protection of the intrinsic hand musculature with broad retractors during transmetacarpal resection in order to avoid iatrogenic muscular or neurovascular injury. Prior cadaveric modeling performed in conjunction with prosthetic and rehabilitation colleagues at our institution determined that a minimum of 3 cm transmetacarpal resection from the MCP joint should be performed to allow for optimal prosthesis fit. Often following resection at this level, the diaphysis of the metacarpals is prominent dorsally, given the loss of the transverse intermetacarpal ligament and their natural bow; therefore, beveling of the remaining distal edge of the metacarpals is recommended to avoid bony prominence.

The donor DI is next transferred to the dorsum of either adjacent metacarpal and secured to the periosteum using 3-0 vicryl suture. Most often,

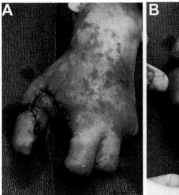
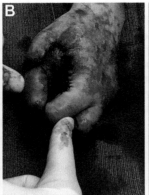
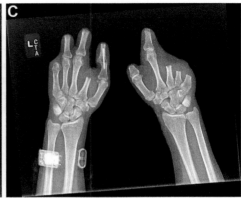

Fig. 3. (A–C) Multiple digit amputations with loss of thumb length to allow for adequate pinch function can be treated with partial heterotopic digit transfer to supplement the available tissue. In the case presented, an on-top plasty of the index finger was performed to achieve adequate length of both digits to allow for satisfactory pinch.

we use the second and fourth DI for control of the long and ring fingers, respectively. Typically, the hypothenar musculature and first DI are present and are preferentially used for signal control of small finger and index finger flexion, respectively. When the hypothenar musculature is absent or insufficient, the third VI or fourth lumbrical can be mobilized to provide signal for small finger flexion. Because all of the intrinsic hand muscles serve as natural MCP flexors, independent, individual digital flexion is highly intuitive following these transfers.

The volar plate and flexor tendon sheath of the involved digits are next mobilized and rotated into the space vacated by the transferred interossei. The volar plate and flexor tendon sheath are sutured to the extrinsic extensor mechanism to create a soft tissue barrier between transferred intrinsic muscles, which prevents unwanted myoelectric cross-talk. Wounds are closed in a tension-free manner with nonabsorbable suture. Suction drains are generally not used, however may be used at the treating surgeon's discretion. The wound is dressed in sterile soft dressings and a bulky soft compressive wrap.

PROSTHESIS USE AND REHABILITATION

Patients are seen in follow-up at 2 weeks postoperatively, at which time sutures are typically removed. Because the transferred muscles are subcutaneous and still innervated, palpable muscle contraction is present immediately. If there is any question as to the function of the transferred muscles, surface EMG testing can be performed at this time. Edema control and exercises to strengthen the transferred intrinsic muscles are initiated at this time. Typically, around 8 to

10 weeks, once the soft tissues and volume have stabilized, the initial mold for the prosthesis is taken. The final prosthesis is typically completed and available for use by 4 to 6 months postoperatively.

Because the control is so intuitive, individual digital prosthetic control can be achieved without significant training (Video 3). We find occupational therapy to be valuable after the Starfish Procedure to maximize strengthening and endurance of the transferred muscles as well as to become proficient with prosthetic use. Our patients typically use the prosthesis on average 8 to 12 hours per day including activities ranging from simple activities of daily living to running a weed eater.

Several opportunities for improvement in prosthesis use following this procedure have been observed in the short- to midterm follow-up. Given the frequency and duration that the transferred interossei are asked to contract, relative to their in vivo recruitment in the unaffected hand, early fatigability and subsequent reduced signal amplitude was observed in the early phases of rehabilitation. This gradual signal amplitude reduction during sustained contractions resulted in loss of sustained digital flexion, allowing the digitals to release at undesirable timepoints. As a result, increased emphasis has been placed on the initiation of early conditioning programs under the supervision of a qualified hand therapist to achieve the requisite muscle endurance for prolonged periods of prosthesis use. The need for a locked-grasp function not requiring sustained signal input was also identified, and modifications to the prostheses were made, which allow for patients to perform a "double contraction" to produce a close and lock grasp of all digits. This allows patients to rest the transferred muscles while the grip is locked, and a simple repeat "double contraction" enables release or opening of the digits. The ability to create sustained grip function with only brief periods of muscle activity required allows for the completion of high-demand activities that would otherwise pose a significant challenge if continuous signal was required. These adaptations furthered patient's abilities to use their prosthetic hands for a variety of tasks throughout the day.

DISCUSSION

The advent of targeted muscle reinnervation (TMR) has shown promising results in improving neuroma-related pain, phantom limb pain, and limb function in proximal upper extremity amputations (transradial, transhumeral, shoulder disarticulation).[30–32] Kuiken and colleagues presented promising early results in both prosthesis adoption and functional outcomes in the use of multifunctional myoelectric prostheses in transhumeral level amputees who underwent TMR.[33] TMR at the transradial level has demonstrated improvements in neuroma-related pain, as well as intuitive myoelectric prosthesis control in several series.[32,34] The use of TMR distal to the radiocarpal level remains quite limited. Elmaraghi and colleagues published a series of 2 patients who underwent TMR for management of postamputation pain control rather than provision of EMG signal for myoelectric prosthesis control as is performed in the proximal upper extremity.[35]

The Starfish Procedure is presently the only method of achieving individual digital control of a myoelectric partial hand prosthesis. We have found a very high rate of utilization likely due to

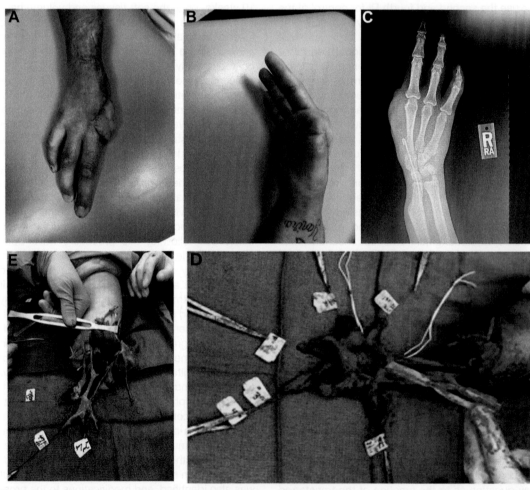

Fig. 4. (*A–E*) Clinical and radiographic appearance of a right hand having undergone prior thumb and index finger amputations with split-thickness skin grafting of a residual radial-sided soft tissue defect. As a result of residual stiffness and limited function the patient elected to proceed with transradial amputation and pedicled Starfish transfers. Figures D and E depict the skeletonized intrinsic musculature, along with their accompanying neurovascular pedicles, as well as the deep palmar arch at the time of transfer.

the intuitive nature of the control. This principle of salvaging innervated muscles during any level amputation is critical, and we refer to this as the Starfish principle. In 2 cases to date, we have had patients with either loss of all digits or completely nonfunctional digits remaining with functional interossei present. Both patients requested forearm level amputation for better prosthetic options. Because the interossei were present and viable, the entire deep arch along with the nerve and blood supply to one interossei muscle per digit (as well as the thenar muscles) was able to be reflected into the forearm at the time of the amputation, and this has allowed individual, distinct signals for all 5 digits to be obtained, which otherwise would not have been possible (**Fig. 4**).

Similarly, the Starfish principle can be applied in the setting of a very proximal forearm level amputation in which the joint is unable to be salvaged. Any flexor-pronator or extensor-supinator muscle that is still viable can be transferred into the residual limb at the time of amputation, thus providing additional signals for myoelectric control.

Fortunately, complications have been rare with this procedure. The most common complication has been wound dehiscence distally when inadequate tissue was present for closure along the distal edge of the wound. Fashioning excess distal skin when possible, potentially even using fillet flaps when needed, can help minimize this complication. To date, all 20 of our cases have generated functioning signals in every transferred muscle, although injury to a neurovascular pedicle remains a concern. Careful attention to the proximal dissection when separating the interossei is critical.

Soft tissue coverage for patients with partial hand amputations also merits discussion. It has become our preference to always use the thinnest possible coverage option in all cases of partial hand amputation. Primary closure is of course the goal always, but when coverage needs are present, we prefer split-thickness skin graft (STSG) when possible or dermal substitutes followed by STSG when necessary. If greater coverage is needed, a radial forearm fascial flap is desirable. Despite concerns for wound breakdown with thin coverage, we have not found this to be the case. Traditional free flaps, groin flaps, and other bulky flaps render prosthetic fitting virtually impossible, and even with extensive debulking, often meaningful prosthetic function is unachievable.

FUTURE DIRECTIONS

Long-term data regarding prosthesis rejection, functional outcomes, and patient-reported outcomes will provide further clarity regarding the durability of the improvements observed in the short-term follow-up currently available. Advanced pattern recognition programs based on individual patient needs may provide for prolonged periods of prosthesis use, as the device integrates more seamlessly with the patient's required activities of daily living. The use of cortical mapping and neural interface systems that allow for central nervous system control of upper extremity prosthesis remains promising, but the investigation of these devices remains ongoing and no commercial option is currently available to patients.[36,37]

SUMMARY

Functional rehabilitation after partial hand amputation is multifactorial. Understanding the occupational and avocational needs of each patient is paramount in providing treatment options, which will maximize their function and quality of life. For those patients with partial hand level amputation who would benefit from the use of myoelectric prosthetic digits for enhanced prehensile function, the Starfish Procedure provides muscle transfers that allow for the generation of intuitively controlled EMG signals for individual digital control with minimal myoelectric cross-talk. Thoughtful preoperative planning allows for creation of multiple sources of high-quality myoelectric signal in a single operation, which does not require microsurgery, providing for wide applicability to hand surgeons of all backgrounds.

CLINICS CARE POINTS

- Functional outcomes following partial hand, or functionally equivalent level, amputations remain a challenge, given the difficulties experienced by patients in completion of both fine motor and power grasp tasks.
- Myoelectric digital control in patients with partial hand amputations remains challenging due to the lack of availability of intuitive EMG signals for prosthesis control.
- The Starfish Procedure allows for the transfer of functioning intrinsic musculature to create sources of EMG signals capable of individual digital control with a prosthesis. This novel transfer method allows for creation of high-quality signals with minimal myoelectric cross-talk.
- Given the lack of microsurgery or other advanced surgical techniques required, this

- procedure remains a viable option for hand surgeons of multiple training backgrounds.
- The intuitive nature of the transfers performed allows for rapid prosthesis adoption and use by patients, which may allow for increased functional use and decreased rates of prosthesis rejection relative to historical controls.

DISCLOSURE

B.J. Loeffler and R.G. Gaston are Hanger Clinic and Checkpoint Surgical consultants.

SUPPLEMENTARY DATA

Supplementary data related to this article can be found online at https://doi.org/10.1016/j.hcl.2021.04.007.

REFERENCES

1. Weinzweig N, Sharzer LA, Starker I. Replantation and revascularization at the transmetacarpal level: long-term functional results. J Hand Surg Am 1996; 21(5):877–83.
2. Paavilainen P, Nietosvaara Y, Tikkinen KA, et al. Long-term results of transmetacarpal replantation. J Plast Reconstr Aesthet Surg 2007;60(7):704–9.
3. Gerostathopoulos N, Efstathopoulos D, Misitzis D, et al. Mid-palm replantation. Long-term results. Acta Orthop Scand Suppl 1995;264:9–11.
4. Chung KC, Yoon AP, Malay S, et al. Patient-reported and functional outcomes after revision amputation and replantation of digit amputations: the FRANCHISE multicenter international retrospective cohort study. JAMA Surg 2019;154(7):637–46.
5. Tosti R, Eberlin KR. "Damage control" hand surgery: evaluation and emergency management of the mangled hand. Hand Clin 2018;34(1):17–26.
6. Wallace CG, Wei FC. Posttraumatic finger reconstruction with microsurgical transplantation of toes. Hand Clin 2007;23(1):117–28.
7. Kotkansalo T, Vilkki SK, Elo P. The functional results of post-traumatic metacarpal hand reconstruction with microvascular toe transfers. J Hand Surg Eur Vol 2009;34(6):730–42.
8. Venkatramani H, Bhardwaj P, Sierakowski A, et al. Functional outcomes of post-traumatic metacarpal hand reconstruction with free toe-to-hand transfer. Indian J Plast Surg 2016;49(1):16–25.
9. Williamson JS, Manktelow RT, Kelly L, et al. Toe-to-finger transfer for post-traumatic reconstruction of the fingerless hand. Can J Surg 2001;44(4):275–83.
10. Waljee JF, Chung KC. Toe-to-hand transfer: evolving indications and relevant outcomes. J Hand Surg Am 2013;38(7):1431–4.
11. Kvernmo HD, Tsai TM. Posttraumatic reconstruction of the hand–a retrospective review of 87 toe-to-hand transfers compared with an earlier report. J Hand Surg Am 2011;36(7):1176–81.
12. Chang NJ, Chang JT, Hsu CC, et al. Heterotopic vascularized joint transfer in mutilating hand injuries. Ann Plast Surg 2016;76(Suppl 1):S1–7.
13. Dean BJF, Branford-White H, Giele H, et al. Management and outcome of acral soft-tissue sarcomas. Bone Joint J 2018;100-B(11):1518–23.
14. Puhaindran ME, Steensma MR, Athanasian EA. Partial hand preservation for large soft tissue sarcomas of the hand. J Hand Surg Am 2010;35(2):291–5.
15. Landry GJ, Mostul CJ, Ahn DS, et al. Causes and outcomes of finger ischemia in hospitalized patients in the intensive care unit. J Vasc Surg 2018;68(5):1499–504.
16. Newbury A, Harper KD, Trionfo A, et al. Why not life and limb? vasopressor use in intensive care unit patients the cause of acute limb ischemia. Hand (N Y) 2020;15(2):177–84.
17. Jung KJ, Nho JH, Cho HK, et al. Amputation of multiple limbs caused by use of inotropics: Case report, a report of 4 cases. Medicine (Baltimore) 2018; 97(5):e9800.
18. Delarosa M, Gaston RG, Loeffler B, et al. Team approach: modern-day prostheses in the mangled hand. JBJS Rev 2019;7(7):e6.
19. Pierrie SN, Gaston RG, Loeffler BJ. Current concepts in upper-extremity amputation. J Hand Surg Am 2018;43(7):657–67.
20. Wright TW, Hagen AD, Wood MB. Prosthetic usage in major upper extremity amputations. J Hand Surg Am 1995;20(4):619–22.
21. Bhaskaranand K, Bhat AK, Acharya KN. Prosthetic rehabilitation in traumatic upper limb amputees (an Indian perspective). Arch Orthop Trauma Surg 2003;123(7):363–6.
22. Otto IA, Kon M, Schuurman AH, et al. Replantation versus Prosthetic Fitting in Traumatic Arm Amputations: A Systematic Review. PLoS One 2015;10(9): e0137729.
23. Farina D, Jiang N, Rehbaum H, et al. The extraction of neural information from the surface EMG for the control of upper-limb prostheses: emerging avenues and challenges. IEEE Trans Neural Syst Rehabil Eng 2014;22(4):797–809.
24. De Luca CJ, Merletti R. Surface myoelectric signal cross-talk among muscles of the leg. Electroencephalogr Clin Neurophysiol 1988;69(6):568–75.
25. Imbinto I, Peccia C, Controzzi M, et al. Treatment of the partial hand amputation: an engineering perspective. IEEE Rev Biomed Eng 2016;9:32–48.
26. Tenore FV, Ramos A, Fahmy A, et al. Decoding of individuated finger movements using surface electromyography. IEEE Trans Biomed Eng 2009;56(5):1427–34.

27. Atzori M, Muller H. Control capabilities of myoelectric robotic prostheses by hand amputees: a scientific research and market overview. Front Syst Neurosci 2015;9:162.

28. Gaston RG, Bracey JW, Tait MA, et al. A novel muscle transfer for independent digital control of a myoelectric prosthesis: the starfish procedure. J Hand Surg Am 2019;44(2):163.e1-5.

29. Woo SH. Practical tips to improve efficiency and success in upper limb replantation. Plast Reconstr Surg 2019;144(5):878e–911e.

30. Dumanian GA, Ko JH, O'Shaughnessy KD, et al. Targeted reinnervation for transhumeral amputees: current surgical technique and update on results. Plast Reconstr Surg 2009;124(3):863–9.

31. Hargrove LJ, Miller LA, Turner K, et al. Myoelectric pattern recognition outperforms direct control for transhumeral amputees with targeted muscle reinnervation: a randomized clinical trial. Sci Rep 2017;7(1):13840.

32. Pierrie SN, Gaston RG, Loeffler BJ. Targeted muscle reinnervation for prosthesis optimization and neuroma management in the setting of transradial amputation. J Hand Surg Am 2019;44(6):525.e1-8.

33. Kuiken TA, Li G, Lock BA, et al. Targeted muscle reinnervation for real-time myoelectric control of multifunction artificial arms. JAMA 2009;301(6):619–28.

34. Morgan EN, Kyle Potter B, Souza JM, et al. Targeted muscle reinnervation for transradial amputation: description of operative technique. Tech Hand Up Extrem Surg 2016;20(4):166–71.

35. Elmaraghi S, Albano NJ, Israel JS, et al. Targeted muscle reinnervation in the hand: treatment and prevention of pain after ray amputation. J Hand Surg Am 2019;45(9):884.e1-e6.

36. Ajiboye AB, Willett FR, Young DR, et al. Restoration of reaching and grasping movements through brain-controlled muscle stimulation in a person with tetraplegia: a proof-of-concept demonstration. Lancet 2017;389(10081):1821–30.

37. Fukuma R, Yanagisawa T, Saitoh Y, et al. Real-time control of a neuroprosthetic hand by magnetoencephalographic signals from paralysed patients. Sci Rep 2016;6:21781.

Recommendations for the Successful Implementation of Upper Limb Prosthetic Technology

Deanna H. Gates, PhD[a],*, Susannah M. Engdahl, PhD[b], Alicia Davis, CPO[c]

KEYWORDS

- Limb loss • Amputation • Prosthetic control • Outcomes • Upper limb

KEY POINTS

- Numerous types of prostheses are available to people with limb loss, some offering multiple degrees of freedom, including different grasp patterns and wrist and elbow movement.
- Advanced surgical approaches, such as targeted muscle reinnervation, regenerative peripheral nerve interfaces, and osseointegration, have the potential to improve upper limb prosthetic control, intuitiveness, comfort, and sensory feedback.
- Integrating patient desires into the prosthetic design is a key component to patient satisfaction.
- Multidisciplinary care teams should be used in the planning of amputation surgery and rehabilitation care postamputation to maximize patient outcomes.

INTRODUCTION

Over the past 50 years, there has been an enormous investment in improving upper limb prosthetic technology. Despite the advancements that have been made, between 23% and 53% of people with upper limb loss abandon prosthesis use,[1,2] and even some of those who use their prostheses heavily report being dissatisfied with them.[3] There are several barriers to the successful adoption of upper limb prostheses, including the perceived limitations in comfort and function of current technology.[4] Patients or clinicians may identify technology that they think would be beneficial, but are often limited in their ability to obtain health care coverage because of the lack of quantitative outcomes demonstrating effectiveness of one prosthetic component over another. The patient may also not be an appropriate candidate for this technology because of his or her residual limb characteristics. Many of these barriers become more pronounced with new prosthetic technology because they often require that patients have specific surgical procedures at the time of or after amputation. Additionally, few new devices developed and presented in the research community are translated into commercial products available to individuals with limb loss.[5] This may be caused by the small market-size for upper limb prostheses, the complexity of the medical device approval process, high development costs,[5] or lack of patient interest in new approaches. This review focuses on the potential barriers and offers solutions to encourage the widespread dissemination and acceptance of new technology, thus maximizing patient outcomes.

[a] School of Kinesiology, University of Michigan, 830 N. University Avenue, Ann Arbor, MI 48109, USA; [b] Department of Bioengineering, George Mason University, 4400 University Drive, MS 1J7, Fairfax, VA 22030, USA; [c] University of Michigan Orthotics and Prosthetics Center, 2850 South Industrial Highway, Suite 400, Ann Arbor, MI 48104, USA
* Corresponding author.
E-mail address: gatesd@umich.edu

Hand Clin 37 (2021) 457–466
https://doi.org/10.1016/j.hcl.2021.05.007
0749-0712/21/© 2021 Elsevier Inc. All rights reserved.

BARRIERS TO ACCEPTANCE OF COMMERCIALLY AVAILABLE PROSTHETIC TECHNOLOGY

There are three categories of active upper limb prostheses, differentiated by their control strategies. Body-powered prostheses are mechanical devices that translate the motion of one body segment (ie, scapula) to the motion of an end-effector through a cable. Myoelectric devices are externally powered (battery) prostheses controlled using surface electromyography (EMG) signals recorded from the residual limb. Finally, hybrid prostheses combine body-powered and electric components to control multiple joints. Currently, there is little empirical evidence to suggest that either body-powered or myoelectric prostheses provide a significant functional advantage over the other.[6,7] However, each of these devices have advantages and disadvantages in terms of perceived comfort and function. For example, a recent literature review found that people abandon body-powered prostheses predominantly for lack of comfort, but some also report difficulty of control, or failure caused by cable breakage.[4] Myoelectric prostheses are reportedly abandoned because of weight, lack of durability, slow response speeds, lack of sensory feedback, and difficulty controlling the prosthesis.[4]

Over the past decade, there have been several advances in myoelectric hands and their control strategies. These devices have been improved from direct control of a single degree of freedom (open/close),[8] to control of complex, multiarticulated hands, such as the Bebionic and Michelangelo from Ottobock (Duderstadt, Germany), the iLimb (Ossur, Reykjavik, Iceland), TASKA hand (Fillauer, Chattanooga, TN), Vincent hand (Vincent Systems, Weingarten, Germany), and the LUKE arm (Mobias Bionics, Manchester, NH). The technical capabilities of different multiarticulated hands are detailed in two recent literature reviews.[9,10] Although these devices significantly increase the degrees of freedom of movement, current commercial systems continue to be limited to only a few independent surface EMG signals that can be recorded from the residual limb. They can also be unintuitive and slow to operate because they are controlled sequentially (eg, grip selection, and then open-close).[10] Although all the fingers move on these hands, it is not yet possible for users to control the fingers independently. Instead, the user selects the grasp patterns using EMG triggers, by pressing a button or using gesture control recorded via sensors in the prosthesis, or blue-tooth chips attached to specific objects.[11] One possible option to manage control of multiple grasp patterns is by adding a pattern recognition system, such as Coapt,[12] MyoPlus,[13] or Sense.[14] In these systems, specific signal characteristics are extracted from up to eight pairs of EMG sensors and can enable users to select, on average, between three and six grasps.[10]

There are several barriers to widespread use of myoelectric prostheses. First, these devices are significantly more expensive than body-powered prostheses and may not be covered by insurance. To justify the need for advanced prosthetic technology, prosthetists must work closely with the physician and occupational therapist to determine if the patient would benefit from myoelectric control and verify the patient has the physical and cognitive ability to learn how to use this technology. Various factors, such as residual limb length, availability of residual innervated muscles and the ability to voluntarily contract these muscles for EMG signals to control the prosthesis, and the environment where the prosthesis will be used are all factors in selecting a myoelectric prosthesis. Determining if the patient will be a successful myoelectric user is exceptionally challenging given the lack of objective outcomes research in this area to suggest that myoelectric control or multiarticulated hands offer significant functional benefits. The lack of outcomes is likely caused by the small population with upper limb amputation (~41,000 people in the United States), the heterogeneous nature of the population, and that multiarticulated prosthetic hands, in particular, have only been available commercially since 2007. The use of these hands can also be limited by their weight, which makes them fatiguing to use and can cause pain from the load placed on the residual limb from the prosthetic socket. Alternative socket designs may help alleviate this weight through more direct loading of the residual bone.[15] However, there are limited studies to support the effects of different socket designs on comfort. As mentioned, improvements to the control of the device are added through commercial pattern recognition systems, but not without significant additional costs. These systems can integrate with existing technology, allowing the prosthetist to combine end-effectors, wrist rotation units, and control systems to customize the device for each patient. However, this approach may not be optimal for many patients because it requires increased initial patient training and frequent recalibration because of movement of the limb in the socket.[16]

BARRIERS TO SUCCESSFUL CLINICAL MANAGEMENT OF PATIENTS WITH UPPER LIMB LOSS

Given the wide variety of prosthetic options, it is imperative that the rehabilitation team works together to determine the optimal prosthetic components for a given patient. The choice of prosthetic options is limited by the state of the limb resulting from the trauma and/or amputation surgery, and the type of prosthesis the patient's insurance company will reimburse. Ideally, prosthetic options would be discussed as part of a multidisciplinary patient care team, or a "group of diverse clinicians who communicate with each other regularly about the care of a defined group of patients and participate in that care."[17] It is well-established that the use of multidisciplinary, in-hospital teams improves patient outcomes, limits adverse events, and improves patient and employee satisfaction.[18,19] Nowhere is this more evident than in the operating room where the surgical team is highly interdependent. As such, the patient's outcome is often determined more by how well the team is able to communicate with mutual respect for each person's skill set than by the specific skill set of any one individual.

Although this approach is effective in most surgical settings, it is typically not adopted in the case of upper extremity amputation. Prosthetists are unfortunately not often an intrinsic part of the initial patient care team, despite being the subspecialists who are ultimately responsible for the design and creation of the patient's prosthesis. One of the main reasons for this lack of interaction between the surgeon and prosthetist is that only 2% of the prosthetists in the United States work in hospital settings.[20] Additionally, the low rate of upper limb loss, combined with the fact that 70% of all upper limb amputations are unplanned[21] (eg, 80% of amputations in men aged 15–45 are caused by trauma[22]), means that there is often no time to engage the prosthetists who are not on site. In contrast, surgeons who regularly conduct lower extremity amputations, most of which are caused by disease, are often afforded the opportunity to formulate a plan of care in coordination with physiatrists, prosthetists, and physical therapists. This multidisciplinary patient care team can then discuss such factors as optimal limb amputation length, patient insurance, and patient occupation and interests, and inviting the patient's input regarding his/her desires and expectations regarding prosthetic rehabilitation.

The following cases highlight the importance of a multidisciplinary team that works together to balance the surgical requirements with the biomechanics of the prosthesis and the patient's needs. By discussing prosthetic options before surgery, including the forces transmitted to the residual limb during activities of daily living, the surgeon may be able to modify the surgical approach to facilitate prosthetic rehabilitation. This is an important consideration because surgeons are often unaware of emerging prosthetic technology, what health care insurances will reimburse, and the physical space required for componentry to optimally restore limb function and symmetry with the contralateral limb. A lack of input from the prosthetist may result in residual limb lengths that are too long to accommodate prosthetic componentry or too short to tolerate the added biomechanical forces of the prosthesis. Without this important feedback, the surgeon and patient may develop unrealistic expectations regarding realistic outcomes for prosthetic restoration. Ultimately, the patient may achieve suboptimal outcomes, often leading to prosthetic abandonment.

In the first case, a patient developed right hand necrosis secondary to sepsis. The necrotic tissue was excised, leaving only the fifth metacarpal intact, resulting in an incomplete transmetacarpal amputation (**Fig. 1**A,B). Prosthetic management of this amputation type does not allow for a socket to be donned, nor does it allow for a prosthesis to be of equal limb length to that of the contralateral side. Although the prosthetist was able to fabricate a type of prosthosis (orthotic device with prosthetic prehension; see **Fig. 1**C,D), the patient's outcome was less than optimal. The patient was not able to use the wrist because of scar tissue impeding motion and the limited surface area on the remaining metacarpal was insufficient to withstand the significant surface pressure of the prosthesis while participating in activities of daily living. Although the patient eventually was able to use the prosthosis, a wrist disarticulation or slightly more proximal amputation would have rendered improved prosthetic rehabilitation by allowing the patient and prosthetist a greater variety of prosthetic options. In particular, it may have been possible to include a prosthetic wrist (for pronation and supination and possibly flexion) or myoelectric components for greater prehension capabilities, including multiple grasp patterns and increased grip forces. Additionally, a total contact prosthetic socket interface would yield greater comfort, function, and limb length symmetry.

In the second case, a patient sustained a work-related crush injury at his midforearm with extensive soft tissue damage and bone fragmentation (**Fig. 2**A). The surgical team worked to preserve the elbow joint and create a short transradial amputation with the thinking that this patient would be

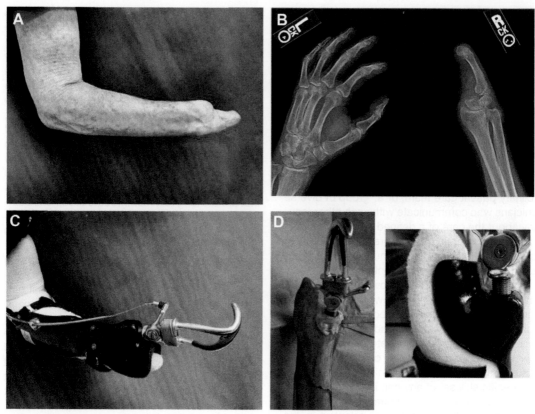

Fig. 1. (*A*) Photograph and (*B*) radiograph of a patient residual limb postamputation surgery. (*C*) Body-powered prosthosis that was made to accommodate the remaining metacarpal of the residual hand after amputation surgery. (*D*) The prosthosis was modified approximately 1-year postamputation to improve comfort and fit around the residual hand.

able to use a myoelectric prosthesis. Part of the surgical process to save the ulna and the elbow joint was to screw the pieces of the ulna together for healing (see **Fig. 2**B). Because of the lack of soft tissue coverage, the screw became prominent once the edema reduced and the prosthesis was a failure because of pain at the site of the screw. Looking closely at the radius, the distal cut bone was not beveled and therefore caused pain when it made contact with the prosthetic socket during elbow flexion. Although the patient had several prosthetic sockets and complete prostheses fabricated by three different prosthetists, in 6 years he has still not been able to wear a prosthesis comfortably.

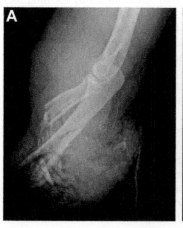
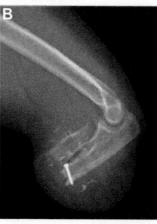

Fig. 2. Radiographs of a patient's upper limb pre (*A*) and post (*B*) surgical intervention. The screw added to stabilize the bone prevented the patient from wearing a prosthesis comfortably.

Another important barrier to clinical management of patients with upper limb loss is a lack of rehabilitation or prosthetic training. Clinicians believe that prosthetic training, defined as practical training in the use of a prosthesis together with a professional,[23] is an important aspect of improving functionality and device usage.[4] Unfortunately, in a survey of people with upper limb loss, only 69% reported receiving any type of training, and only 63% believed that this training was sufficient.[23] Lack of prosthetic training was also cited as a contributing factor for device abandonment.[23] One reason for the lack of training may be the lack of coverage through health care insurance. When training is provided, its success depends on the clinician's experience with that specific type of prosthesis and the patient's willingness to fully engage in training. Given the complexity of new multiarticulated hands and pattern recognition systems, the clinician must become specialized. To maximize a patient's functional benefits and discourage frustration and device fatigue, insurance companies should support the procurement of the device and training with a prosthetist or occupational therapist who specializes in the care of people with upper limb absence.

One can look to US military facilities for an example of how a multidisciplinary team can work effectively to improve prosthetic patient outcomes. All patient care disciplines are colocated in these facilities, promoting the multidisciplinary team approach. Furthermore, the US Veterans Administration and the Department of Defense have created a clinical practice guideline that includes an algorithm for postamputation care throughout the perioperative phase, preprosthetic phase, prosthetic training phase, and the lifelong care phase.[24] Thus, the care team can follow a set protocol for each patient to maximize his or her outcomes.

EMERGING APPROACHES TO IMPROVE PROSTHETIC CONTROL AND COMFORT

Given the high rates of abandonment and dissatisfaction, recent research has focused on the development of new surgical approaches and technologies to improve the comfort, fit, and function of prostheses. All newly developed approaches are intended for use with myoelectric devices, because they are the current state of the art in the field. Because these are new approaches (<10 years) and many have only been explored in the research laboratory, it is currently unclear how they may improve satisfaction and device use.

There are several approaches that have been developed to address the issues of lack of independent EMG signals that are recorded from the residual limb and long training times required by pattern recognition approaches. Several noninvasive options have been proposed to increase the number of control signals by measuring the movement of other body segments through inertial measurement units,[25] sensorized insoles,[26] or electrogoniometers,[27] or sensing residual muscle activity using ultrasound.[28] Numerous advancements have also been made in surgical approaches to enhance prosthetic control. Implantable myoelectric sensors can be chronically implanted into residual muscles via minimally invasive surgical techniques,[29] or sensors are placed directly into the nerve itself.[30] Alternatively, surgeons have developed novel approaches to harness volitional signals from transected peripheral nerves within the residual limb after amputation. In targeted muscle reinnervation (TMR), the surgeon transfers the residual peripheral nerves to denervated muscles near the amputated limb.[31] These signals can then be captured using a grid of surface electrodes, processed using pattern recognition, and used to control a multidegree of freedom prosthesis.[31] To create a regenerative peripheral nerve interface (RPNI), the surgeon attaches an autologous free muscle graft to the end of a residual nerve.[32] As the nerve grows, it reinnervates the free muscle graft, which undergoes a predictable sequence of revascularization and regeneration. EMG signals from RPNIs demonstrate high signal-to-noise ratios when interrogated with needle electrodes or when indwelling bipolar electrodes are surgically implanted within them.[33] These signals have been used to successfully control a multiarticular prosthetic hand, including individual, independent movement of all fingers including the thumb.[33]

Similar surgical approaches can be exploited to provide sensory feedback to the user. Traditional myoelectric prostheses provide some feedback to the user through vision, auditory cues, vibrations, or pressure transmitted through the socket,[34] and potentially kinesthetic feedback through muscle contraction to activate the myoelectric control. To enhance the feedback provided, several research groups have developed systems to provide artificial sensation. Sensory feedback is delivered either via sensory substitution techniques (eg, mechanically vibrating the skin of the residual limb in response to a stimulus)[35] or by targeting sensory organs (eg, modality matching). Researchers have successfully elicited proprioception and tactile sensations through direct neural stimulation with an invasive electrode,[36] electrical stimulation of RPNIs,[37] and pressure stimulation of the reinnervated skin after TMR surgery.[38] This work is limited to a few individuals, mostly in controlled laboratory environments, although a few have been extended to take home trials.[38]

Finally, some efforts have been made toward forgoing the socket altogether and instead directly attaching the prosthesis to residual bone in a surgical procedure known as osseointegration. This procedure has been used for attachment of artificial limbs in Europe since 1990,[39] but has only recently become available in the United States. This approach can also be combined with surgical control and feedback techniques through systems, such as the e-OPRA Implant System (Integrum, Molndal, Sweden), which routes wires from electrodes directly attached to muscles through an osseointegrated implant and out of an abutment. This allows direct electrical connection between the muscle signals and prosthesis,[40] and eliminates the need for more complex wireless transmission. The utility of this approach was demonstrated in a person with a transhumeral amputation and chronically implanted muscle and nerve electrodes for motor control and sensory feedback, respectively.[41] The patient was able to complete activities of daily living with the osseointegrated prosthesis for more than 1 year. Although this technique has great potential, it is not yet part of clinical care because of concerns about infection or implant loosening.

PATIENT INTEREST IN SURGICAL APPROACHES TO IMPROVE PROSTHETIC CONTROL AND COMFORT

With the development of new surgical approaches, it is increasingly important to understand which procedures patients would be willing to undergo to achieve improved comfort and control given the associated surgical risks. In a survey of 232 individuals with upper limb loss, 58% responded that they would be "likely" or "very likely" to try TMR to restore dexterity or touch, 64% would try peripheral nerve implants, and 38% would try cortical interfaces.[42] Similarly, 49% of 808 Veterans with upper limb loss were willing to consider surgery for improved control over finger movements, grasps, or wrist motions.[43] Slightly fewer individuals (42% with unilateral limb loss and 41% with bilateral limb loss) would consider surgery to restore a sense of touch.[43] Only 28% of those with unilateral limb loss and 13% of those with bilateral limb loss were willing to consider osseointegration surgery to avoid the need for prosthetic sockets.[44]

Individuals with upper limb loss anticipate that these surgical approaches will enable a variety of benefits. The most common benefits mentioned during open-ended interviews were lighter prostheses, more comfortable and secure prosthesis attachment, and improved functionality for activities of daily living.[45] For surveyed individuals willing to consider surgery to restore touch or to improve motor control, the most important perceived benefits were device durability, comfort, and the ability to perform more activities.[43] These three benefits were also most important for individuals willing to consider osseointegration surgery.[44]

Despite this recognition of potential benefits, patients are also concerned about the associated medical risks.[46] Long-term medical risks, such as chronic pain or need for device removal because of failure, were most concerning to individuals willing to consider osseointegration,[44] and surgery to restore touch or to improve movement control.[43] Short-term medical risks were more acceptable to all groups.[43,44] Concerns about undergoing additional medical procedures beyond those involved with the initial amputation or experiencing a loss of function in the residual limb were frequently mentioned by participants in a focus group study.[47] Similar concerns are shared by other stakeholders in the limb loss community. Forty-seven surveyed stakeholders (including those with limb loss) reported that their primary concerns about invasive interfaces related to either effectiveness or minimizing medical risks.[48] Those who were concerned about effectiveness tended to cite functionality issues (device reliability, malfunction, training, and time between surgery and use), whereas the others focused more on medical concerns (surgery, infection, device invasiveness, and tissue removal).

Although collectively these findings indicate patients are interested in new surgical approaches, there are several caveats. First, there is considerable diversity in patient opinion. Although some patients have no reservations about undergoing surgery, others are unwilling to consider a potentially risky procedure under any circumstance.[46] Many others report openness to considering surgical approaches as long as they have been proven to be successful.[45,46] Second, patient needs and interests must continue to be evaluated as the technology evolves. Both patients and other stakeholders in the limb loss community have emphasized a desire to delay decision-making until the technology progresses out of the research stages.[47,49] Similarly, stakeholders have acknowledged that it is difficult to prioritize their concerns in a theoretic context without truly knowing which risks and benefits will become reality.[48] As these technologies become increasingly available to participants in research studies and eventually in commercial use, evaluating how they work in real-world settings will be useful in refining patients' opinions.

UPDATING CLINICAL PRACTICE FOR EMERGING TECHNOLOGY

Given the existence of new technology and surgical approaches, it becomes incumbent on clinicians to manage patient expectations given their specific circumstances. As noted previously, this is ideally done as part of a multidisciplinary patient care team focused on preamputation and postamputation plans. Here we highlight a few additional challenges that are created by novel surgical approaches.

For surgeries that include implanting electrodes into the residual muscles, it is imperative that the surgeon has an understanding of the prosthetic device that will be used by the patient. Specifically, the degrees of freedom of the device and its control algorithm will dictate which muscles should serve as inputs to the system. Typically, these prosthetic components are limited in the number of channels they are capable of recording so it is imperative that the input signals are selected appropriately. For example, the surgeon should

work with the prosthetic rehabilitation team to determine if a wrist rotation unit will be included. Motion of the wrist is crucial for orienting the prosthetic hand so that it can interact with objects. However, wrist rotation units are not available with all prostheses and some require substantial space, which cannot be accommodated if the patient has a long residual limb. Without knowing the prosthesis that the patient will be prescribed, the surgeon could potentially place electrodes in muscles that would never be used at the expense of others that may have utility for enhanced function.

Surgical approaches to enhance motor control may also limit the prosthetist's ability to fit the patient with a comfortable, stable prosthetic socket that adequately distributes the load. For operations where electrodes are implanted in residual innervated muscles, the electrodes pass transcutaneously to an external control unit. The socket then needs to be adapted with cutouts to accommodate these wires. For this reason it is imperative that the surgeon knows which area of the skin will be load bearing or subject to compression when the elbow or shoulder bends (**Fig. 3**).

Because this field is evolving at a rapid pace, it is important that all stakeholders involved in the treatment and dissemination of upper limb prosthetic technology stay up to date with current developments in their areas of expertise.

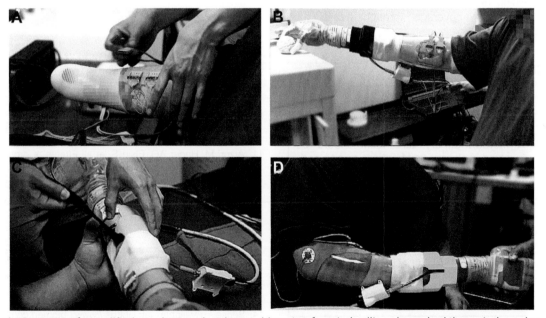

Fig. 3. Image of a modified prosthetic socket that enables wires from indwelling electrodes (*A*) to exit the socket (*B*). A custom three-dimensional printed wrist attachment allowed the wires from the hand unit to exit the wrist attachment and connect to a computer. (*C*) Because of the initial indwelling wires exiting the skin where the socket needed to connect, the research team used a silicone liner with lanyard strap to connect the socket to the patient. (*D*) The modified socket was used to complete functional tasks and activities of daily living.

Multidisciplinary conferences, such as the Myoelectric Controls Symposium, the International Society of Prosthetics and Orthotics, and other national conferences on prosthetic control, can aid in this process by bringing together patients, prosthetists, surgeons, physiatrists, occupational therapists, researchers, and device manufacturers to highlight the latest innovations and evidence-based research on prosthetics.

SUMMARY

We believe that patient outcomes with upper limb prostheses may be maximized with the development of an appropriate multidisciplinary team, updated clinical practice guidelines to reflect emerging technologies, and open dialogue between prosthetic designers, clinicians and patients to promote the development of prostheses that people want to use. This could help alleviate some bottlenecks, help the patients feel more informed about their choices, and allow the patient and care team to develop realistic expectations for potential outcomes. In order for this to become a reality, research should focus on studies quantifying functional outcomes, patient satisfaction, and abandonment rates over extended periods of time using new technology. These studies are necessary, not only for establishing expectations, but also for encouraging clinician interest in providing new technology to their patients and funding their coverage through health care agencies.

CLINICS CARE POINTS

- A multidisciplinary care team should be involved in all aspects of patient care to optimize the patient's potential to use a prosthesis based on their unique needs and goals.
- Patients may require specialized training to become proficient using advanced technology. This should be incorporated into the patient's health care plan.
- There is a critical need for additional outcomes research to promote health care coverage for existing and emerging technologies.

DISCLOSURE

The authors have nothing to disclose.

REFERENCES

1. Biddiss EA, Chau TT. Upper limb prosthesis use and abandonment: a survey of the last 25 years. Prosthet Orthot Int 2007;31(3):236–57.
2. Sugawara AT, Ramos VD, Alfieri FM, et al. Abandonment of assistive products: assessing abandonment levels and factors that impact on it. Disabil Rehabil Assist Technol 2018;13(7):716–23.
3. Davidson J. A survey of the satisfaction of upper limb amputees with their prostheses, their lifestyles, and their abilities. J Hand Ther 2002; 15(1):62–70.
4. Smail LC, Neal C, Wilkins C, et al. Comfort and function remain key factors in upper limb prosthetic abandonment: findings of a scoping review. Disabil Rehabil Assist Technol 2020;1–10.
5. Farina D, Amsuss S. Reflections on the present and future of upper limb prostheses. Expert Rev Med Devices 2016;13(4):321–4.
6. Carey SL, Lura DJ, Highsmith MJ, CP, FAAOP. Differences in myoelectric and body-powered upper-limb prostheses: systematic literature review. J Rehabil Res Dev 2015;52(3):247–62.
7. Carey SL, Lura DJ, Highsmith MJ. Differences in myoelectric and body-powered upper-limb prostheses: systematic literature review. J Prosthet Orthot 2017;29(4S):P4–16.
8. Wurth SM, Hargrove LJ. A real-time comparison between direct control, sequential pattern recognition control and simultaneous pattern recognition control using a Fitts' law style assessment procedure. J Neuroeng Rehabil 2014;11:91.
9. Belter JT, Segil JL, Dollar AM, et al. Mechanical design and performance specifications of anthropomorphic prosthetic hands: a review. J Rehabil Res Dev 2013;50(5):599–618.
10. Atzori M, Muller H. Control capabilities of myoelectric robotic prostheses by hand amputees: a scientific research and market overview. Front Syst Neurosci 2015;9:162.
11. Atzori M, Hager AG, Elsig S, et al. Effects of prosthesis use on the capability to control myoelectric robotic prosthetic hands. Conf Proc IEEE Eng Med Biol Soc 2015;2015:3456–9.
12. CoApt Engineering. Available at: https:// coaptengineering.com. Accessed September 20, 2020.
13. MyoPlus. Available at: https://www.ottobockus.com/prosthetics/upper-limb-prosthetics/solution-overview/myo-plus.html. Accessed September 20, 2020.
14. Sense. Available at: https://www.i-biomed.com/sense.html. Accessed September 20, 2020.
15. Alley RD, Williams TW, Albuquerque MJ, Altobelli DE. Prosthetic sockets stabilized by alternating

areas of tissue compression. J Rehabil Res Dev 2011;48(6–10):679.

16. Resnik LJ, Acluche F, Lieberman Klinger S. User experience of controlling the DEKA Arm with EMG pattern recognition. PLoS One 2018;13(9): e0203987.

17. Wagner EH. The role of patient care teams in chronic disease management. BMJ 2000;320(7234): 569–72.

18. Epstein NE. Multidisciplinary in-hospital teams improve patient outcomes: a review. Surg Neurol Int 2014;5(Suppl 7):S295–303.

19. El Saghir NS, Keating NL, Carlson RW, et al. Tumor boards: optimizing the structure and improving efficiency of multidisciplinary management of patients with cancer worldwide. Am Soc Clin Oncol Educ Book 2014;e461–6.

20. Whiteside S. Practice analysis of certified practitioners in the disciplines of orthotics and prosthetics. In: Alexandria VA, editor. American Board for Certification of Prosthetist. Orthotists & Pedorthotics; 2015.

21. Barmparas G, Inaba K, Teixeira PGR, et al. Epidemiology of post-traumatic limb amputation: a national trauma databank analysis. Am Surg 2010;76(11): 1214–22.

22. Maduri P, Akhondi H. Upper limb amputation. In: StatPearls. Treasure Island, FL. 2021.

23. Østlie K, Lesjø IM, Franklin RJ, et al. Prosthesis rejection in acquired major upper-limb amputees: a population-based survey. Disabil Rehabil Assist Technol 2012;7(4):294–303.

24. Department of Veterans Affairs and Department of Defense. Clinical practice guideline for the management of upper extremity amputation rehabilitation 2014. Available at: https://www.healthquality.va.gov/guidelines/Rehab/UEAR/VADoDCPGManagementofUEAR121614Corrected508.pdf.

25. Resnik L, Klinger SL, Etter K, et al. Controlling a multi-degree of freedom upper limb prosthesis using foot controls: user experience. Disabil Rehabil Assist Technol 2013;9(4):318–29.

26. Carrozza MC, Persichetti A, Laschi C, et al. A wearable biomechatronic interface for controlling robots with voluntary foot movements. IEEE ASME Trans Mechatron 2007;12(1):1–11.

27. Luzzio CC. Controlling an artificial arm with foot movements. Neurorehabil Neural Repair 2000; 14(3):207–12.

28. Dhawan AS, Mukherjee B, Patwardhan S, et al. Proprioceptive sonomyographic control: a novel method for intuitive and proportional control of multiple degrees-of-freedom for individuals with upper extremity limb loss. Sci Rep 2019;9(1):9499.

29. Weir RF, Troyk PR, DeMichele GA, et al. Implantable myoelectric sensors (IMESs) for intramuscular electromyogram recording. IEEE Trans Biomed Eng 2009;56(1):159–71.

30. Clark GA, Ledbetter NM, Warren DJ, et al. Recording sensory and motor information from peripheral nerves with Utah Slanted Electrode Arrays. In: Paper presented at: 2011 Annual international conference of the IEEE Engineering in Medicine and Biology Society. 2011.

31. Kuiken TA, Li G, Lock BA, et al. Targeted muscle reinnervation for real-time myoelectric control of multifunction artificial arms. JAMA 2009;301(6):619–28.

32. Kung TA, Langhals NB, Martin DC, et al. Regenerative peripheral nerve interface viability and signal transduction with an implanted electrode. Plast Reconstr Surg 2014;133(6):1380–94.

33. Vu PP, Vaskov AK, Irwin ZT, et al. A regenerative peripheral nerve interface allows real-time control of an artificial hand in upper limb amputees. Sci Transl Med 2020;12(533):eaay2857.

34. Wijk U, Carlsson I. Forearm amputees' views of prosthesis use and sensory feedback. J Hand Ther 2015;28(3):269–78.

35. Antfolk C, D'Alonzo M, Rosén B, et al. Sensory feedback in upper limb prosthetics. Expert Rev Med Devices 2013;10(1):45–54.

36. Wendelken S, Page DM, Davis T, et al. Restoration of motor control and proprioceptive and cutaneous sensation in humans with prior upper-limb amputation via multiple Utah Slanted Electrode Arrays (USEAs) implanted in residual peripheral arm nerves. J Neuroeng Rehabil 2017;14(1):121.

37. Vu P, Vaskov AK, Irwin ZT, et al. A regenerative peripheral nerve interface for real-time control of an artificial hand. Sci Transl Med 2020;12(533): eaay2857. In Review.

38. Schofield JS, Shell CE, Beckler DT, et al. Long-term home-use of sensory-motor-integrated bidirectional bionic prosthetic arms promotes functional, perceptual, and cognitive changes. Front Neurosci 2020; 14:120.

39. Hagberg K, Branemark R. One hundred patients treated with osseointegrated transfemoral amputation prostheses: rehabilitation perspective. J Rehabil Res Dev 2009;46(3):331–44.

40. Ortiz-Catalan M, Mastinu E, Sassu P, et al. Self-contained neuromusculoskeletal arm prostheses. N Engl J Med 2020;382(18):1732–8.

41. Ortiz-Catalan M, Hakansson B, Branemark R. An osseointegrated human-machine gateway for long-term sensory feedback and motor control of artificial limbs. Sci Transl Med 2014;6(257):257re256.

42. Engdahl SM, Chestek CA, Kelly B, et al. Factors associated with interest in novel interfaces for upper limb prosthesis control. PLoS One 2017;12(8): e0182482.

43. Resnik L, Benz H, Borgia M, et al. Patient perspectives on benefits and risks of implantable interfaces for upper limb prostheses: a national survey. Expert Rev Med Devices 2019;16(6):515–40.

44. Resnik L, Benz H, Borgia M, et al. Patient perspectives on osseointegration: a national survey of veterans with upper limb amputation. PM R 2019;11(12):1261–71.

45. Benz HL, Jia Y, Rose L, et al. Upper extremity prosthesis user perspectives on unmet needs and innovative technology. Conf Proc IEEE Eng Med Biol Soc 2016;2016:287–90.

46. Engdahl SM, Christie BP, Kelly B, et al. Surveying the interest of individuals with upper limb loss in novel prosthetic control techniques. J Neuroeng Rehabil 2015;12:53.

47. Zheng JY, Kalpakjian C, Larraga-Martinez M, et al. Priorities for the design and control of upper limb prostheses: a focus group study. Disabil Health J 2019;12(4):706–11.

48. Janssen EM, Benz HL, Tsai JH, et al. Identifying and prioritizing concerns associated with prosthetic devices for use in a benefit-risk assessment: a mixed-methods approach. Expert Rev Med Devices 2018;15(5):385–98.

49. Kelley MA, Benz H, Engdahl S, et al. Identifying the benefits and risks of emerging integration methods for upper limb prosthetic devices in the United States: an environmental scan. Expert Rev Med Devices 2019;16(7):631–41.

Moving?

Make sure your subscription moves with you!

To notify us of your new address, find your **Clinics Account Number** (located on your mailing label above your name), and contact customer service at:

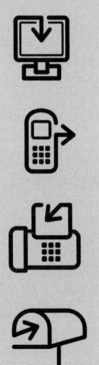

Email: **journalscustomerservice-usa@elsevier.com**

800-654-2452 (subscribers in the U.S. & Canada)
314-447-8871 (subscribers outside of the U.S. & Canada)

Fax number: **314-447-8029**

**Elsevier Health Sciences Division
Subscription Customer Service
3251 Riverport Lane
Maryland Heights, MO 63043**

ELSEVIER

Printed and bound by CPI Group (UK) Ltd, Croydon, CR0 4YY

08/05/2025

01864697-0015